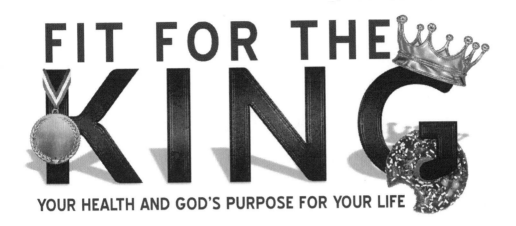

FIT FOR THE KING

YOUR HEALTH AND GOD'S PURPOSE FOR YOUR LIFE

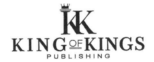

KING OF KINGS
PUBLISHING

DAVID BUSH
WITH JOE TEWELL

David Wishes To Acknowledge

Writing a book is one thing; putting it into eminently readable form is another. I'm very grateful for the team that has come around me to help in this endeavor. My editor, Steve Cooper, my publishing and licensing liaison, John Desaulniers, and my graphics and layout expert Nicole Young have been indispensable in helping make this book a reality.

Many thanks to Joe Tewell, my friend, partner, and contributor to this book. Our long conversations over many years have finally taken form here. Hopefully this is the beginning and not the end.

I owe a debt of gratitude to my pastor, Mike Rose, whose sermon topics in recent years have found their way into some of the chapters of this book.

I appreciate the many people who read early versions for feedback as well as copy editing, including Nikki Jackson and Stephen Bush.

Most importantly, thanks to my wife, Beth, and family who have had to deal with weekly stresses and challenges as I have worked on this book for more than a year. Your help, encouragement, and sacrifices have allowed this to move forward.

Soli Deo Gloria
David Bush
December, 2014

TABLE OF CONTENTS
Introduction

PART FIVE
TRANSFORMATION

INTRODUCTION

For want of a nail, the horseshoe was lost. For want of a horseshoe, the steed was lost. For want of a steed, the message was not delivered. For want of an undelivered message, the war was lost. — Ancient Proverb

"...for truly, I say to you, if you have faith like a grain of mustard seed, you will say to this mountain, 'Move from here to there,' and it will move, and nothing will be impossible for you."
— Jesus in Matthew 17:20

Throughout the writing of this book, I've been confronted time and again with the oversized impact that small, daily body-care decisions have on our overall quality of life, our testimony to others, and, ultimately, our lifespan. I've witnessed the real-life repercussions of practiced habits, and the liberating influence of a right understanding of the gospel.

I saw it again this week. Within a thirty-six-hour period, our cultural and spiritual war with food, inactivity, and personal obsession was played out in the lives of several of my friends and associates.

My first encounter was at a funeral home. Shuffling through the visitation line that queued before a grieving family, I passed by pictures of the deceased chronicling his life journey. There he was playing basketball for the high school varsity team. Another shot captured a college date night with his future wife. Then came the family photos of daddy and toddlers, the week fishing in the mountains, and, finally, Pop in his favorite recliner watching a football game. The photo collage of the passing years revealed a gradually expanding waistline, and it was not lost on those in attendance that the massive heart attack that claimed his life at 56 was earned one meal at a time.

For one of his boys, these precious family memories will be forever eclipsed by the final, terrifying minutes of his father's life as the son tried to revive his father with CPR on the floor of an Iowa barn. For the extended family, the incremental impact of his death will include a premature and unplanned exit from two generations of family farming.

Another encounter came in the office of a former world-class athlete and bi-vocational pastor, who related to me his exasperation at the disconnect he felt between his faith and the state of his family's health. "My wife and I recognized recently that, despite knowing better, we've developed some bad habits as a family," he confessed. "Our kids are in sports, my wife works, and we've fallen into the trap of eating fast food too often because of our crazy schedules. I jump on the kids for all their wasted time in front of the TV, but I'm walking right past a gym every day knowing that, despite my slender build, I'm not as fit as I should be."

The following morning I sat in a coffee shop with a veteran podiatrist talking about the toll our cultural excesses are taking on our bodies. "In the early years of my practice, my days were filled with patients seeking help with corns, bunions, athlete's foot, toenail fungus and plantar warts" he related. "Today, I'm dealing with serious foot issues arising from diabetes and obesity, as well as overuse by marathon runners and ironmen."

A final conversation was with a young woman whose maturing walk with Christ had set her free from a downward spiral of compulsive dieting and anorexia. After years of denial and living in the shadows, she is now counseling other young women with similar struggles, and making God-honoring decisions with her husband in the area of meal preparation and nutrition.

As these stories illustrate, the current of our culture is relentlessly carrying us downstream to a future marked by immobility, inefficiency, costly medical bills, lost opportunities, and lost lives. For the average person, this is a tragedy that is unnecessary and reversible. For the Christian, fighting against this current is just another countercultural mandate of our faith.

Like any work that challenges the prevailing norms of behavior, the contents of this book will provide ample occasion for offense for those who seek it. My goal is not to shame, dispirit, condemn, or marginalize anyone. Neither is it to suggest some monolithic physiological goal that should animate every believer's life. What I hope to accomplish with this book, associated workbooks, and through Inspire™ health conferences is help you understand the significance our physical bodies have in the Kingdom plan and work of God. As I write, "We were created on purpose and for a purpose." This fact, coupled with the assurance that nothing is impossible where Jesus is invited, should inspire each of us to view our lives as a holy trust with eternal value.

Joining me in bringing this book to you is my contributor Joe Tewell, whose life experiences and fitness wisdom I've sought to put into words. I highly value his contributions to this endeavor. A graphic showing a barbell will accompany chapters he has contributed to.

Making health and fitness a priority in your life doesn't equate to a restricted life with fewer options. Pursuing a fit life actually increases your enjoyment and your productivity as you find yourself available for greater accomplishments! May the Holy Spirit guide, direct, convict, and encourage all of us to make sober assessments of our lives and habits, and commit ourselves to lives that are continually transforming to better reflect the image of our King!

David Bush

PART ONE
FIT FOR WORSHIP

CHAPTER 1

REASONABLE WORSHIP

Therefore I urge you, brethren, by the mercies of God, to present your bodies a living and holy sacrifice, acceptable to God, which is your spiritual service of worship. And do not be conformed to this world, but be transformed by the renewing of your mind, so that you may prove what the will of God is, that which is good and acceptable and perfect.
Romans 12:1-2 (NASB)

I'm inviting you to join the Love Revolution. It's not the kind of revolution that is fueled by anger and protest, but one that's motivated by a love for God and others that compels you to think and act differently. Not a revolution against some enemy outside the church, but one that starts inside each of us and overflows to those outside. It's a revolution in what it means to worship God. A revolution animated not by an ideology or legalistic orthodoxy, but of worship in its most practical form. Joining this revolution will be costly, life changing, and well worth the sacrifices it will ask of you.

Simply put, I'm inviting you to join a revolutionary movement to think and act biblically in regard to your physical body. Like the Apostle Paul writing to the believers in Rome, I am writing with both a sense of urgency as well as a desire that you hear God's mercy and grace. At its core, this is a worship revolution the Church must embrace if it is to move beyond the limited and superficial definition of worship it has adopted in our time. This revolution is comprised of ideas as big as body ownership and life purpose, and as small as menu choices and exercise routines.

Since you've made it past the cover of this book, perhaps you have at least a passing interest in health and fitness or are considering some lifestyle changes (or the resolve to stick with those you've already adopted). You also likely have a couple of important questions. First, what relevance does the Bible and worship have in regard to body care issues? Second, what does an unknown Worship Pastor from Iowa have to add to the conversation?

Biblical Relevance

The Bible has a great deal of instruction on this topic, and the purpose of this book is to bring together relevant Scripture and practical, life-giving application. Romans 12:1-2 is a foundational Scripture that provides clear evidence of God's intentional connection of your body and worship. For the follower of Christ, body care is not of secondary importance after worship: *body care is worship*. By body care, I mean cleaning, eating balanced meals and keeping fit. Acknowledging that God owns the rights to your body and moving to a place of surrender, obedience and availability—that's daily, costly worship.

It's also *reasonable worship*. Using the word *therefore* in verse 12:1, Paul is transitioning from the enumeration of God's manifold blessings in the previous eleven chapters to point out that **a lifestyle of physiological worship is the only right and logical response to God's largesse**. In fact, the Greek word that is most often translated *spiritual* or *reasonable* service is *logikos*, from which we get the English word logical.

My Perspective and Goal

Given this clear connection between your reasonable worship and physical surrender, perhaps the perspective of a Worship Pastor can be of some help as we explore God's intentions and purposes for your body. I'm leaving the development of detailed diet, workout, nutritional and recipe books for other authors. In the majority of this volume, I will focus on the arena Paul identifies as the true battlefield for control of your body: the mind. My goal is to allow God's word to renew your mind so, after thinking rightly, you have the tools to act rightly.

As one who's been deeply involved in the Christian music industry and most recently in the growing world of contemporary worship music, I have seen firsthand how worship has been "rebranded" to include only the twenty-minute song set we encounter at our Saturday night or Sunday morning services. Lost is the truth that every aspect of our lives is worship, including stewardship of our physical bodies.

Becoming and remaining physically fit has been a lifelong passion of mine. As a believer in Jesus for over forty years (and a follower of His for something less than that), I've been concerned that my pursuit of fitness is balanced and inspired by a solid scriptural foundation. I've spent years thinking, writing, and speaking about balanced fitness—wondering if other more influential voices in the Christian community would begin to take up the challenge.

Worshipping in a Culture of Extremes

Our culture has increasingly offered two unacceptable alternatives: sedate and consumptive lifestyles or an unhealthy pursuit of all things related to sports and fitness. In the void of biblical teaching and modeling, Christ-followers have generally conformed themselves to the thinking and actions of one of these two dominant cultural trends. Solomon said "without a vision the people are unrestrained" and I believe *unrestrained* characterizes well the faith community today. Believers fall into two unfortunate groups: They are demonstrably more unfit than their secular counterparts or they make an idol out of athletic pursuits.

Our country is in the midst of a health crisis, and I believe it is appropriate for the Church to speak boldly and knowledgably to the issues confronting us as a society. Believers have been instructed in a better way to live, and it's time for us to lead by example. I hope this book will serve to move followers of Jesus to that end.

How to Benefit From This Book

I have organized this material into five parts that are intended to be read and applied sequentially. I present a biblical perspective of your body along with a rationale for pursuing a life of balance and fitness. Nutrition and exercise expert Joe Tewell helps you with practical information about developing a healthy lifestyle. Joe has acquired more licenses and certifications in the area of fitness and nutrition than anyone I know, and has spent a lifetime as a gym owner and personal trainer helping people reach their fitness goals. Our goal is not to prescribe workout or diet absolutes, but to present sound information that focuses on motivations and behaviors that take root in the battleground of your mind. Please avoid the temptation to skip forward. Moving on to practical applications without first understanding the foundation of our approach will undermine our purposes and hold you back from achieving all that's possible as a Christian.

First, you must understand and own the problems we all have with our current approaches to diet and fitness, as well as cast a vision for what worshipful fitness looks like. After Joe and I share our stories and describe how they've informed our approaches to this topic, we'll do the important work of demolishing wrong thinking and actions in the area of nutrition and fitness. From there, we'll help you build a new understanding of your body. You'll then be prepared to embark on a journey of transformation toward becoming the holistic worshipper God desires you to be. You are encouraged to access online help via our website at *www.fit4theking.net.*

Whatever your present physical condition or perspective of health and fitness, this pursuit will almost certainly cost you something. Don't focus on the cost! Turn your thoughts and attention instead to the worthiness of the One who has called you into a loving, grace-saturated worship experience that transcends the pleasures and pursuits of this world. The Old Testament says, *"The eyes of the LORD search the whole earth in order to strengthen those whose hearts are fully committed to him"* 2 Chronicles 16:9 (NLT). My prayer is that after applying what you learn here, you will catch the notice of God as one who is giving a worthy sacrifice of worship through stewardship of your body.

If the Church begins to lead in the area of body care, there will be not only revolutionary changes in the depth and fervency of our worship, but also a tangible change in our witness to those outside the body of Christ who are desperate to experience fit and healthy lifestyles that work.

Live Like That

Sometimes I think
What will people say of me
When I'm only just a memory
When I'm home where my soul belongs?

Was I love
When no one else would show up?
Was I Jesus to the least of us
Was my worship more than just a song?

Am I proof
That You are who you say You are
That grace can really change our heart
Do I live like Your love is true?

People pass
And even if they don't know my name
Is there evidence that I've been changed
When they see me, do they see You?

I want to live like that
And give it all I have
So that everything I say and do
Points to You

If love is who I am
Then this is where I'll stand
Recklessly abandoned
Never holding back

I want to live like that

Words and Music by David Frey, Ben McDonald and Ben Glover
© 2011 DaySpring Music LLC/Ariose Music Group, Inc./9TOne Songs
Used by permission

CHAPTER 2
WORSHIP WARS

From my perch on the auditorium platform, I could make out the features of most who are attending this morning's worship service, despite the room's dimmed lights. As the Pastor of Worship Ministries for the church I serve, this vantage point has become familiar. I recognize most of the faces, along with the seats they occupy. Many of their stories are familiar as well, as I've been at least a peripheral part of the triumphs, tragedies and challenges they've experienced through our years worshipping together.

On a typical Sunday, my focus is squarely on building a personal and corporate connection with the living God. Today, however, I'm looking out at the assembled worshippers through a different filter. I've just begun writing the book you now hold in your hands, and for some reason this particular morning I'm unable to distinguish their physiological journeys from their spiritual ones.

I've asked them to stand as we begin our time of worship through singing. On tap this morning are songs of praise and aspiration, including a well-worn favorite:

Hungry

Hungry I come to You for I know You satisfy
I am empty, but I know Your love does not run dry
So I wait for You, So I wait for You
I'm falling on my knees
Offering all of me
Jesus, You're all this heart is living for …

Words and Music by Kathryn Scott ©1999 Vineyard Songs (UK/Eire)
Used by permission

Near the back, in the center of the row, Carl has his eyes closed and his hands raised as he sings from memory. From all outward appearances, Carl is affirming long-held convictions. But the 100+ excess pounds he's carried around for 30 years seem to indicate he's been hungry for satisfaction beyond what he experiences with the Lord. Because of the burden his insatiable hunger placed on his extremities, he had a double knee replacement last year, and just a month ago he'd nearly died of a massive heart attack. He was saved by an alert neighbor. In the weeks following he appeared to have dropped some weight and was on the road to recovery, but in recent weeks the tide appeared to change yet again as his brush with death receded and his usual living patterns returned.

Across the aisle was Stuart, who was making a rare appearance at worship. Stuart is an avid triathlete and coach of his kid's soccer team. I remember visiting his home and seeing his study wall, which had been dedicated to displaying medals, framed photos and trophies he'd acquired through the years. Between training, Sunday games, practices and competitions, Stu found it hard to be consistently involved at church. His fist was pumping, however, as our next worship chorus (apparently one of his favorites) continued our theme:

Run

You are God, You are holy
History is Your story
You who was, and is, and Who forever will be
God, we live for Your glory!
We will run all together with hearts aflame
With a fire that can't be tamed
Our God, all glory to Your Name—Jesus!

Words and Music by Joel Houston ©2008 Hillsong Music Publishing
Used by permission

Worshipping in front of Stuart was Candace, who had struggled for years with obesity. Months ago Candace requested prayer for an "unnamed surgical procedure," had disappeared for a couple of months, and was now back wearing clothes that no longer fit her shrinking physique. Her lips formed the words to a chorus she seemed to know well:

Inside Out

A thousand times I've failed, still Your mercy remains
And should I stumble again, still I'm caught in Your grace
Everlasting, Your light will shine when all else fades

Never-ending, Your glory goes beyond all fame
In my heart and my soul
Lord I give You control
Consume me from the inside out
Let justice and praise become my embrace
To love You from the inside out

Words and Music by Joel Houston ©2005 Hillsong Music Publishing
Used by permission

A quick scan of another section revealed a recovering anorexic, an avid runner who had just completed his twelfth marathon, a middle-aged Deacon who had just begun daily insulin injections for his adult-onset diabetes and a gentleman who was having a hard time joining in the worship, distracted as he seemed to be by the low-cut blouse and enhanced bust line of a fellow parishioner.

I'm taken aback not only by my decidedly non-worshipful thought process, but by the pain, hurt and baggage that is on public display. The issues people are dealing with are manifesting themselves, in a variety of ways, in their bodies. I'm also struck by the apparent disconnect many in our congregation seem to have between what they say and what they do. Has our worship become a fifteen-minute song set instead of an expression of our devotion and commitment to God?

The ironic blindness, needs and brokenness of our congregation's physical state are screaming at me this morning. Admittedly, these have been songs of aspiration—we are *aspiring* to become living examples of what these lyrics portray—but the potential for hypocrisy seems great. I can't see hearts, discern motives nor understand extenuating circumstances, but by all outward appearances average Christians have issues with body care that need addressing. We seem to be tottering on the edge of idolatry. As believers in Christ, we are obliged to pursue *discipleship*. But are we?

The Discipleship Connection

I've just returned from a national discipleship conference sponsored by the Verge Network (*vergenetwork.org*). Leaders in the Missional Church Movement remind us of the centrality of following Jesus and being Jesus as we engage our families, communities, co-workers, and neighbors. As I absorbed the scene in my own church, I was struck by how consumer-driven and irrelevant we as the Church have become. Our expectations are too often that our church leadership will provide the religious goods and services that meet our felt needs—all packaged in an enjoyable context. Rather than joining with other life-raft rowers called to a tempest-tossed world, we are like luxury liners in dry dock waiting for a favorable high tide that never comes.

At the Verge Network conference, dozens of national speakers and presenters of both sexes, of all ages, and of many ethnicities appeared physically fit. They were "on mission," available, and engaged. This was a stunning contrast to what I encounter at most churches, where tired, over-scheduled, overfed, and complacent parishioners gather weekly to "do church."

I am fully aware that speaking with any sense of authority on issues of lifestyle, fitness and body consciousness is fraught with the potential for misunderstanding. Many will undoubtedly assume the premise itself is judgmental and superficial. But I'm compelled by love and concern to address a visible epidemic in the Church with repercussions most have never considered. If you love someone, you risk the potential for offense to tell the truth. *"Friends Don't Let Friends Drive Drunk"* is a well-accepted practice because we understand the potential tragedy awaiting those who through pressure or cowardice don't demand the car keys. Maybe we need Christian worship slogans, such as *"Friends don't let friends defile the temple"* or *"Friends don't let friends persist in idolatry of diet and fitness."* This is a pervasive spiritual and worship issue that can no longer be ignored.

A Healthy Motivation For Health And Fitness

There are countless books discussing health, fitness and diet on the market, most authored by doctors who have a new discovery that will "revolutionize" the way you eat, a celebrity seeking to extend their shelf life by trading on their access to plastic surgeons, or fitness experts who practically live in gyms. Their roadmaps for health are often driven by consumption of hard-to-find or exclusive foods, the purchase of special equipment, or impractical fitness regimens. The Christian market has been treated to recent entries, including one advocating we eat only what Jesus ate (perfect for all residents of Galilee).

While some of these volumes are a pure money grab hatched by savvy marketers, many of these books and programs contain sound information. But a quick survey of the human landscape makes it clear that, with a few notable exceptions, most of these plans don't morph into lasting lifestyle changes. Perhaps this is because so few address key issues that condemn these diets and routines to failure. *Jumping into a diet or fitness program without proper motivation and a healthy perspective of your body will only lead to frustration and failure as you chase an elusive cultural ideal.* Let's face it, if you don't have God's perspective about your physical body, your purpose for living, and a biblical rationale for pursuing fitness, what good are revolutionary workout regimens and "superfoods"?

A Culture of Extremes

As I previously noted, we live in a culture that is pushing us toward one of two extremes. On one hand, we idolize health and fitness, body image and beauty. The pursuit of all things *me*. On the other hand, we've become bloated caricatures of human beings who seem to have lost all sense of self-control and self-respect. Cloaked at times beneath words of self-deprecation this, too, is the pursuit of all things *me*. The same bookstores, magazine racks, and Kindles that are overflowing with offers of help for our dietary and sedentary hangovers also offer countless opportunities to worship at the altars of health, beauty, and extreme fitness. During a time when our society becomes increasingly immobile and drug dependent, there is a large and growing community of bodybuilders, triathletes, and amateur sports-league players whose lives revolve around their next workout or meals from blenders. A society that is pressing the limits of self-destruction and self-absorption in every conceivable area is at its bipolar best when it comes to our physical state.

As believers, it shouldn't surprise us that the culture is staggering about in a physiological fog. But how is it that these two secular forces became epidemic in the church? Is it even possible to find a lifestyle of sustainable balance between the relentless pull of these two carnal forces?

Statistics relating to our nation's increasing obesity and declining health make this trend stunningly clear.

• *More than a third of Americans are obese today; 69 percent are overweight or obese; 74 percent of men are overweight or obese; 8 percent of women are extremely obese. [1]*

• *In the early 1970's 6 percent of U.S. teenagers were obese. By 2007, this number had jumped to 18 percent. Plus, 12 percent of children ages two to five are obese. [2]*

• *In 2004 16 percent of active military personnel were obese and in 2005 27 percent of military candidates were too overweight to be considered for service. Obesity is currently the leading cause of discharge from and disqualification for military service. [3]*

• *In the 1950s per capita consumption of cheese was almost eight pounds per year. In 2000 it was nearly thirty pounds per year. [4]*

- *Since 2000, hip and knee replacement surgeries have nearly doubled, to over 1 million procedures a year. Surgeries for those under fifty-nine years of age have dramatically escalated and are significantly influenced by obesity. [5]*

- *In 1993, 17,000 bariatric (weight loss) surgeries were performed. About 220,000 such surgeries are now performed annually. [6]*

- *The obesity epidemic has brought sharply higher rates of high blood pressure, heart attacks, stroke, type 2 diabetes, nonalcoholic fatty liver disease and osteoarthritis. [7]*

- *Unless there are dramatic changes in the current trends, researchers indicate that 42 percent of adult Americans will be obese by 2030. [8]*

Imagine what the obesity rate would be if we were not undergoing over 500,000 liposuction procedures and 220,000 weight loss surgeries per year! Statistics are cold, impersonal things. Remember that behind all these distressing numbers are people who need answers, alternatives, and inspiration to start in a new direction.

But the statistics showing our pursuit of physical beauty and obsessive fitness also reveal a lot about our society.

- *The number of surgical and non-surgical cosmetic procedures for women has increased by 252 percent in seventeen years. In the same period, procedures for men increased 106 percent. [9]*

- *10 billion was spent on cosmetic procedures in 2011. [10]*

- *Over 1 million American adults have used anabolic steroids, and it has become an increasing problem among high school athletes. [11]*

- *Membership in USA Triathlon was 128,000 in 1999. By 2013 there were over 550,000 members. [12]*

- *Retail sales in sports nutrition rose to over $21 billion in 2011. [13]*

• With sales pushing $5 billion a year, tanning salons outnumber McDonald's restaurants in the U.S. This growth comes amidst a barrage of media publicizing the dangers of tanning beds and their link with growing levels of skin cancer. [14]

• The 17,000 health clubs open in 2000 grew to nearly 30,000 in 2008. [15]

These figures are all derived during a period of time when the U.S. was experiencing its worst financial downturn since the Great Depression of the 1930s. What we're spending on convenience food, medical care, cosmetics, cosmetic surgical procedures, and extreme fitness pursuits has become such a priority that we will incur debt, defer the mortgage payment, and cut back on charitable giving in order to acquire what we think we need or deserve.

A Problem In The Pews

This is not happening in secret. As I compiled these figures, I was keenly aware of the hundreds of people I know that are represented in these statistics, These are friends, family members, neighbors, co-workers and fellow believers— even myself.

I wish I could affirm that the Church possesses a reputation for balancing these two cultural polarities, but in engaging these growing trends the phrase "The Silence of the Lambs" would be appropriate. In one of the most potent cultural trends of the past two decades, we have allowed the conversation to be molded by product and service marketers, celebrities, and, increasingly, the federal government. In my 35 years of adult participation in church services, I've heard one sermon on what the Bible says about our physical bodies as it pertains to health and fitness—and I gave that sermon. When was the last time you heard a message on gluttony? A message addressing vanity?

In many areas we may, as the Church, represent a restraining force in our society regarding destructive habits, practices, and behaviors. In the arena of food and fitness, however, Christians may actually be leading our culture into the gastronomical abyss. Despite possessing ultimate Truth, we have suspended logic in this area and have, through willful ignorance or intellectual and spiritual disobedience, determined that neither God's laws nor the laws of cause and effect apply to what we put in our mouths or how we address our personal health.

"America is becoming known as a nation of gluttony and obesity, and churches are a feeding ground for this problem," says Purdue University sociology professor

Ken Ferraro who has studied religion and body-weight issues since the early 1990s. *"If religious leaders and organizations neglect this issue, they will contribute to an epidemic that will cost the health-care system millions of dollars and reduce the quality of life for many parishioners."* [16]

Perhaps this book can serve to elevate that critical conversation in the Body of Christ. Pastor and author John Piper speaks to the dangers of cultural capitulation when he writes:

"Until we waken to our darkened spiritual condition, we live in sync with 'the present evil age' and the ruler of it (Ephesians 2:2). Without knowing it, we were lackeys of the Devil. What felt like freedom was bondage. The Bible speaks straight to twenty-first-century fads, fun and addictions when it says, 'They promise them freedom, but they themselves are slaves of corruption. For whatever overcomes a person, to that he is enslaved' (2 Peter 2:19). The resounding cry of freedom in the Bible is, 'Do not be conformed to this world, but be transformed by the renewal of your mind' (Romans 12:2)." [17]

This is not a diet book; you don't need another diet. After all, 95 percent of all dieters will regain their lost weight within five years, and a substantial number of dieters will eventually develop eating disorders. [18] Of the over 600 diets that are commercially marketed today [19], few are designed to create healthy, balanced, *sustainable* lifestyles. Rarer still are books that address the critical need to demolish wrong thinking and motivations, while establishing an appropriate foundation for understanding God's perspective on our bodies and fitness.

As anxious as Joe and I are to see a more fit society, we're also distressed to see the unbridled passion for fitness that characterizes so many of our lives. As wonderful as it is to see people embrace a healthy lifestyle, we are increasingly uncomfortable with the priority we see this given, and the enormous amounts of time and energy that are expended pursuing what can easily become a self-focused cultural ideal.

Our worship is practically expressed through where we spend our time and money, and through what consumes our minds. By this definition, far too many of us are worshipping ourselves. Both extremes I've been describing are incompatible with a life lived in submission to and for the glory of the King.

A Question of Motivation

On one level, it's understandable why those identifying themselves as Christians (and pastors) are 10 percent fatter than the average North American and 50 percent more likely to become obese by middle age than nonbelievers.[20] Consider the motivations marketed to those who want to change their physical appearance.

- "You give so much of yourself to others; it's time to do something for yourself!"
- "You'll never compete with younger workers if you don't lose thirty pounds!"
- "After your divorce, you need to get ready to get 'back on the market!'"
- "Lose forty pounds and show him/her what he/she lost!"
- "Bikini season is just around the corner!"

Most of these rationales for change contain elements many Christians would find questionable. So how does the Christian become motivated and empowered to make necessary changes to their thinking and their actions in regard to their physical bodies if what the world is peddling rings hollow?

Joe and I hope to present a compelling biblical motivation for change through what's presented in these pages. We hope you will develop a personal conviction that caring properly for your body is a critical part of what it means to be a disciple of Jesus Christ.

A Balanced Approach

What Joe and I present here (and in our online tools) comes from decades of real-life experience in the Church and in the fitness and Nutrition industries, a litany of personal mistakes and wrong priorities, a multi-year investigation into biblical teaching regarding our physical bodies, seminars, and sermons on this topic. We have also sought guidance from the Holy Spirit.

We're not newcomers to this. No wispy twenty-somethings trading on their youthful metabolism here. Between us, we've logged over 100 years of living. Our schedules are filled with career obligations, kid's activities, college visits, church activities, commutes and car pools. We hear the call of a comfortable lounge chair as loudly as anyone and recognize that the commercials for products promising to reverse declining testosterone levels are targeted toward us. We feel the lure of fast food restaurants and convenience foods as keenly as anyone else. We have, however, developed deep-rooted convictions that have carried us through many life stages and helped us navigate through the morass of cultural misinformation that confronts us all on a daily basis.

Are you tired of diets and confused by volumes of contradictions? Are you frustrated and discouraged with how you look and feel? Do you ever wonder if you've crossed the line from a healthy self-image to self-obsessed vanity? Is there a biblical dichotomy between your spiritual and physical lives? Are you curious how the Great Commandment and the Great Commission should inform your perspective on diet and fitness? Are you looking for biblical motivation to stick with a fitness plan? Are you interested in a fitness plan that is *sustainable*? Are you hungry for balanced thinking and acting in an unbalanced culture?

If your answer to some or all of these questions is "yes", then *Fit For The King* has been written for you!

And we urge you, brothers, admonish the idle, encourage the fainthearted, help the weak, be patient with them all. 1 Thessalonians 5:14 (ESV)

1. Centers For Disease Control NTCS Data Brief No. 82. January 2012.
2. Centers for Disease Control, "FastFacts."
3. *Mission:Readiness, Too Fat To Fight* (Washington, D.C.). Mission: Readiness, 2010, accessed at *www.missionreadiness.org/2010/toofattofight/*. *Unfit For Service: The Implications of Rising Obesity for U.S. Military Recruitment*. John Cowley and Johanna Catherine Mclean. Health Economics 21, no. 11 (2012) 1348 – 66.
4. *Profiling Food Consumption In America* U.S. Dept. of Agriculture Factbook.
5. *The Relationship Between Obesity and The Age At Which Hip and Knee Replacement Is Undertaken*. M. Changulani, Y. Kalairajah, T. Peel, RE Field. March 2008 National Institutes of Health Publication. OECD:Library:Statistics 2011 derived from Centers For Disease Control Statistics.
6. Bariatric Surgery Maintains, Doesn't Gain. Victoria Stagg Elliot April 23, 2012.
7. *The Economic Impact of Obesity in the United States*. Ross Hammond and Ruth Levine. Brookings Institution. *Amednews.com*.
8. Eric Finkelstein, American Journal of Preventative Medicine Vol. 42, Issue 6. June 2012 Pgs 563-570.
9. *Association Between Obesity and Psychiatric Disorders in the US Adult Population*. Simon, Von Korff, Saunders, Miglioretti, Crane, van Belle, Kessler. July 2006 Journal of the American Medical Association.
10. *Cosmetic Surgery: 15 Years of Facts and Figures* American Society for Aesthetic Plastic Surgery. May 3, 2012.
11. Centers For Disease Control survey: Substance Abuse and Mental Health Services Administration May 16, 2012.
12. *Growth In the Sport of Triathlon Fueled by Committed, Motivated Athletes* According to *Active Network Findings* Active Network Press Release Sept 21, 2010; USA Triathlon. org Demographics.
13. *The Next Chapter In Sports Nutrition*. Janica Lane. *NeutriceuticalWorld.com* May 2012.
14. *Burned By Health Warnings, Defiant Tanning Industry Assails Doctors 'Sun Scare' Conspiracy*. Bridget Hubber. *Fairwarning.org* August 23, 2012.
15. *Fitness Industry Analysis*. Andrew Weber. *Franchisehelp.com* 2013.
16. Purdue University News. August 24, 2006.
17. *50 Reasons Why Jesus Came To Die* Dr. John Piper.
18. *Eating Disorder Statistics*. National Association of Anorexia Nervosa and Associated Disorders 10-year Study, 2000.
19. *www.everydiet.org/completelist*.
20. *Study Finds Link Between Religion, Obesity*. Michael De Groote. *Deseret News*. April 5, 2011.

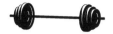

CHAPTER 3

BUILDING YOUR FUTURE: THE NECESSITY OF URGENCY

This book is about your future. Rather than being an incidental issue that can be tucked away for a more convenient time, how you address your health *right now* will have ramifications on your financial, spiritual, relational, and medical life story. When we're young, there is no sense of urgency about this issue of physiological investment. We generally feel good, live without physical limitations, and are focused on the immediate. A wise person, however, will regularly raise their eyes to search the horizon. This practice will inform your present and reveal if the life story you're currently writing will be one you want to live in the future.

What kind of life story are you writing?

Perhaps you are in the early chapters, where the characters are being introduced and the setting is being described. Maybe you're in the middle where the plot is being developed and a crisis is presented. Or perhaps you're near the end, when resolution brings a sense of satisfaction.

Wherever you are, there are opportunities you can grasp *right now* that can help assure your story unfolds with the purpose, vitality, and the fruitfulness you and your Creator desire.

One of the hardest visions to cast today is a vision of the *future*. For all of us, each day is filled with so much activity, we feel justified pride in just getting successfully through each day. This myopic tendency, however, has become very costly. Financial guru Dave Ramsey helps many begin thinking about their financial futures. His countercultural admonition is to "live like no one else, so that someday you can live like no one else." His appeal seeks to prepare us financially for a truth that cannot be emphasized enough: ***For most people, the window of greatest impact on their families, their businesses, their churches, and their world will be between the ages of fifty and seventy.***

It is in these two decades that your accumulated wisdom and experience, your financial resources, your relational capital, and your increasingly flexible schedules can be leveraged for maximum impact. For the passionate follower of Christ, this is the stage of life when you will undoubtedly have the greatest impact for the Kingdom of God.

Health, fitness, and nutritional decisions and patterns you're pursuing *right now* are major factors influencing your future life story. Will you be:

— a grandmother who can join in her grandchildren's adventures or who never makes those memories,

— a father who is actively engaged with his children's lives and activities or who has to watch from the sidelines,

— an empty-nest couple with the physical and financial ability to invest in others or a couple that spends all their time and resources on doctor's appointments and prescriptions,

— a man or woman forced to rely solely on a broken and dysfunctional health care system as you age,

— a person experiencing a world that is expanding in opportunity or slowly shrinking,

— a believer still able to say "yes" or "no" to opportunity?

Make no mistake, there is a physical dimension to each of the answers you've given. I know far too many people whose self-inflicted health issues make a major impact in their lives before they reach even their fiftieth birthdays.

Are you looking at your future now and asking, "What do I do now?" You don't want to end up like Jimmy Stewart's character in "It's A Wonderful Life," living in a physiological Pottersville because of the way you are handling the opportunities that come your way today. Regardless of your physical condition, there are wise steps you can take immediately that will make oversized impact on the future of your health.

Since David has emphasized the need to deal with some foundational issues before moving forward with a body-care plan, I'm going to give you twelve things you must *stop* doing if you want to clear the deck for future success. If you're not prepared to address my "Dirty Dozen" list, it is likely you're not yet ready to reexamine food and fitness, and the tangible way each can make an impact on your family, your vocation, and your faith walk.

JOE'S DIRTY DOZEN

1. <u>Stop wasting time in front of the TV.</u> It's quite possible that you will have to make a choice between your health and watching every "must see" series or improving your score on your video game system.

2. <u>Stop dehydrating yourself while drinking empty calories.</u> Regular and diet sodas may be the single biggest dietary villains stealing your future.

3. <u>Stop depriving yourself of sleep.</u> You need a minimum of six-and-one-half to seven hours per night. And no, you're not wired differently.

4. <u>Stop snacking after 8 p.m.</u> Nothing good happens between you and the fridge after 8 p.m.

5. <u>Stop acting like you're indestructible.</u> This applies both to the workaholic and the fitness junkie.

6. <u>Stop making prescription drugs your first alternative.</u> How do you suppose people survived prior to the 1970s? All our drugs have not made us a healthier nation.

7. <u>Stop comparing yourself to other people</u>. Have you discovered yet that this is a joy and gratitude stealer?

8. <u>Stop obsessing about everything you eat.</u> Food is an unworthy object of our worship, and is a merciless taskmaster.

9. <u>Stop abusing alcohol, tobacco, and drugs.</u> Pretty basic, I know, but it has to be said. Seek out professional help now if this is an issue for you.

10. <u>Stop falling for the lie that healthy choices are convenient or that physical transformation is easy.</u> The "quick fix" doesn't exist and likely does more damage than good.

11. <u>Stop exercising ownership rights to your body.</u> You weren't your idea, you're not in charge, and you make a terrible boss.

12. <u>Stop making excuses.</u> They aren't any more legitimate just because they come from you.

FIT FOR THE KING

I live in the same culture as you. I recognize that our consumer-driven society constantly seeks to focus us on the immediate. In the midst of this tyranny of the urgent, we neglect some extremely important things. These include living wills, estate planning, hugging our kids, and actually praying for those to whom we promise our support.

There also exists the proper and necessary urgency to plan for your future legacy. What you accomplish and experience in your life and invest in others will be greatly impacted by your health. This book is intended to be a roadmap that will help you on your journey. Of course, you are free to postpone your serious need to address the fitness path you are on now, just as you are free to take the unwise step of erecting roadblocks that will detour you from God's potential for your life.

Or you can decide to get started *right now*.

CHAPTER 4

FIT FOR THE KING: WHAT DOES IT TAKE?

Now may the God of peace himself sanctify you completely, and may your whole spirit and soul and body be kept blameless at the coming of our Lord Jesus Christ. He who calls you is faithful; he will surely do it.
1 Thessalonians 5:23-24 (ESV)

As a Worship Pastor, I'm continually faced with the challenge of helping people see that our worship of Jesus is not constrained by music, much less the twenty minutes we might spend worshipping in a weekend church service. While the Old and New Testaments make it clear that music and singing are critical modes of worship, they make it equally clear that God desires far more from us than a passionately delivered hymn or worship chorus. He desires and rightfully expects ***all of us—spirit, mind and body.***

God is our Father. We are His children. Jesus is the King of Kings. We are His subjects. While our church culture and modern translations have done their best to show us the softer side of our Savior, at our own peril we forget that our relationship with Jesus is not as one of His peers. He may be the Good Shepherd, but He's still the shepherd—not part of the flock. He is the Master; we are the slaves. It's no surprise that the Lord has expectations for our lives, particularly that we should follow Him and obey His will. My first radio single, "All About You," speaks to this important basic perspective on life.

All About You

I have played the fool
I fancied myself as the man in the middle
Pretending the fate of the ages revolves around me …
Yet I walk on a borrowed stage
Without strength for a single day

27

Every breath a gift of Your sovereign grace …
Where do I go … What do I do …
I've asked myself, now I'm asking You
I'm standing still, so make me move
It's not about me … it's all about You

Words and Music by David Bush ©2003 Rhyme of the Times Publishing
Used by permission

If we're free agents to do as we please with our lives—and our bodies—then much of this book is irrelevant. If, however, we are created purposefully and have been brought into a relationship with Jesus for the glory of God and **His** Kingdom purposes, our response of worship can't help but be holistic.

God has created us mind, body, and spirit. We have been taught extensively about what it means to love and obey God with our spirits.

Dr. April Crommett, associate professor of exercise science at Cedarville University, rightly notes our teaching has been incomplete: *"In the health and wellness industry, the philosophical debate has morphed into three corners: mind, body, and spirit. The mind and body are cared for in spas, fitness centers, and hospitals, and the spirit ... well, we don't do 'spirit.' And if you were to peek inside the church doors, you may conclude that the church doesn't do 'mind or body.'"* [1]

While the world (and even the Church) seems to segregate our lives into spheres, believing God may care about some more than others, the Bible reminds us that God doesn't see us this way. Our Creator is longing for worship that encompasses the totality of our lives. A familiar Old Testament admonition that is affirmed by Jesus in Mark's Gospel as being the most important pursuit in life is:

"You shall love the Lord your God with all your heart, and with all your
soul, and with all your mind, and with all your strength"
Mark 12:30 (ESV).

Pretty all-inclusive. In addition to our voices, our entire beings are to be surrendered to God for His use, purposes and glory.

Heart = Our control center—the epicenter of our will and motives.

Soul = Our eternal self-consciousness, innermost being, personality, priorities.

Mind = Thought capacity/gatekeeping of input—rational thought and knowledge.

Strength = Bodily powers, physical capacity, influence, time, health, longevity.

No matter your church affiliation or traditions, your pursuit of God's glory all comes down to the heart—the *motivation* for why you do what you do. Are you singing *to the Lord* or just parroting words the congregation is singing? Are you accumulating knowledge at school or work *for the glory and use of the Lord* or because you want to impress people, land a good job, or because you have nothing better to do after high school? Do you train and condition your body **as an act of worship** or primarily to attract more dates, impress people, burn off nervous energy, or socialize with people?

Becoming Fit For The King

In four words, the title of this book speaks to the activity you pursue as well as the motivation. "Fitness" is the goal. "For The King" is the motivation. *In Western society, developing a healthy lifestyle for the right reason is indeed a conscious act of worship.* In a culture that is pulling you toward either complacency and indulgence or obsession with self, taking up the challenge of being *Fit For The King* is a very practical way to love God with your heart, soul, mind, and strength.

Following His affirmation of the Greatest Commandment, Jesus says that there is a second, critical pursuit that should be central to your life as His follower: *"You shall love your neighbor as yourself."*

Loving God with all you are and *allowing Him to love others through you* sums up the entire Gospel. This is what pleases Him. This is what brings Him glory. This is true worship. In a phrase, this means:

> *Being "Fit For The King" means being physically available to love God completely, let Him love others through you, and accomplish all He desires with you for His glory.*

The key word here is *available*. Are you *physically available to respond* and follow Jesus where He leads? This might sound strange as our availability to God is most often couched in terms of **time** as in *will you take the time to attend the weekly Bible Study? Or will you make the time to reach out to your neighbor?* As we move through this topic together, however, I believe you will see that a wrong approach to diet and fitness puts us in a position of being "unavailable" to consider many things God is calling us to do. By following our culture, you put up barriers hindering your ability to obey, serve, and glorify your King and build His Kingdom.

Perhaps you were assuming I would present a height/weight chart or a "godly BMI range" that would direct your thinking. You may be a bit confused by the definition of *Fit For The King* that I gave above. Maybe it would be helpful if

I describe availability in financial terms. I'll use an example drawn from some financial decisions my wife, Beth, and I have made.

Financial worship

Beth and I were married in our mid-twenties and bought a condominium in my native Southern California in the late 1980s. After a year of marriage, we accepted an invitation to join a family business in Beth's home state of Iowa, and because of the large disparity in housing costs, were able to trade up to a much larger home in a nice Des Moines suburb. With no kids, two well-paid jobs, and some investments, we were in a great place financially.

In those early days, Beth and I would take early evening walks around our neighborhood looking at other people's houses. We noticed the well-kept landscaping, the expansive decks, outdoor furniture, boats, motor coaches, and late model cars. Despite the nice things we had, we couldn't help but notice that many of our neighbors had accumulated substantially more nice things than we had. We especially liked the houses on the cul-de-sac nearby that backed up to the country club. There was one specific house we loved that was within our means, but buying it would have meant taking out a considerably larger mortgage.

I remember walking around our childless house looking at all our furniture, the crystal, and china we'd received as gifts at our wedding. I was thinking how nice our furnishings would look—along with a bunch of new furniture—in that house backing up to the seventh tee. At the same time there was another competing Voice that said, *"You can buy that house and fill it up with stuff. But if you do, will you still be available for Me and My plans?"* I realized we were at something of a crossroads in our walk with Christ. This decision had nothing to do with attending Sunday services or a mid-week Bible study. It went beyond our ability to tithe to the church. The purchase Beth and I were considering had implications regarding our future **availability** to love Him through our obedience as well as our **availability** to let Him love others through us. This was a **worship** decision.

Nearly twenty-five years have passed since wrestling with that financial decision. Instead of moving up, we decided to move down. This decision remains one of the most critically important worship decisions we've ever made. After praying and talking about our situation, Beth and I felt the Lord leading us to take a pass on the golf-course house so we could buy Beth's grandparent's empty and deteriorating sixty-year-old home on the "blue collar" side of town. Instead of taking on a larger mortgage and filling up a larger home with more stuff, we remodeled an older home and were able to become completely debt-free about ten years later. The binding weight of debt was gone—and that made us *available*.

I was available to say "yes" when my pastor asked me to leave my executive position and accept a part-time church salary leading an evangelism initiative. I was available to partially fund four original music projects, which led to ministry on radio and at concerts nationwide. Later I accepted a worship position at my church, which paid a fraction of what I would have been making in my former career.

Beth was available to leave her job so she could work part-time at home as God blessed us with a family. She was able to say "yes" when she felt God leading her to homeschool our kids. She was available to help provide leadership for many youth, women's ministries, and activities at our church because she didn't have to leave home for an 8-to-5 job. Beyond tithing, together we've responded to many special financial needs both inside and outside of our church body because we are freed from debt and are *available to respond* when God prompts us to worship Him financially in some way.

Physically available to worship

From our story of financial stewardship, you can see how choices we've made regarding our finances have had a long-lasting and incremental impact on our ability to obey when God has asked us to respond. There have been a few big decisions, but most of our availability has come from monthly, weekly, and daily decisions to maximize our availability. These decisions have almost always run counter to what our culture believes would be best for us. Look at the mess our society is in financially, however, and you can see what a blessing it has been to live counter-culturally and to be unusually available for God in many areas of His Kingdom work. *Avoiding the extremes of our culture has helped us find a biblical balance in every aspect of our lives, including our physical bodies. It's been a blessing.*

So let's return to our defining phrase and see if it makes more sense now:

Being "Fit For The King" means being <u>physically available</u> to love God completely, let Him love others through you, and accomplish all He desires with you for His glory.

Perhaps you've never considered yourself physically "unavailable" to God or your neighbor. After all, you go to church on Sunday and Wednesday nights and even help at the annual church cleanup day. You don't think of yourself as being vain or self-obsessed, but being physically available goes much deeper than that. Glorifying God in your body means more as well. Meeting the needs or your spouse, your children, and your non-family neighbors asks still more of you.

Loving your Lord God with all your heart, soul, mind, and strength, and loving your neighbor as yourself remains the all-encompassing goal of the true worshipper. Being *Fit For The King* is a crucial component of obeying this greatest Commandment.

1.   *Cedarville* Magazine. April Crommet. Fall, 2013 Pg 21.

PART TWO

PUTTING OUR CARDS ON THE TABLE

CHAPTER 5
DAVID'S STORY

There are a few times in a man's life when he searches his heart to make sense of things that don't. These are introspective moments when the soul's longing for transcendent order has to give way to realities on the ground. It happens when you and doctors stand helpless by the bed of your critically ill child. It happens when you walk out of your employer's offices with a pink slip in your hand. Or when one of your parents dies.

Today it's happening for me.

Every man's story is indelibly marked by their relationship with their father. The last chapter of that story with my father has just been written, and now that it's completed, I'm trying to gain perspective that will inform my future.

I've just been escorted into the viewing room at a mortuary in Laguna Hills, California, to say goodbye to Dad. For some reason I thought my solitary visit would provide closure for a relationship that had, due to both geography and relational atrophy, grown increasingly distant. In his seventy-nine years, he had experienced soaring highs and debilitating lows. Sixty years were filled with fruitful labor, but Dad merely endured the last nineteen. He was at peace now, his physical crucible completed. So I said goodbye, and in my grief, shed tears of gratitude and regret. I was comforted to know he was free from the mortal chains that hold all of us captive. Also, to be honest, I was saddened that we'd been saying goodbye to each other for a long time.

Raised in the South Central Los Angeles city of Compton in the 1950's, my dad, Richard Bush, knew nothing of the stereotypical life popularized by the television shows *Leave It To Beaver* and *Happy Days*. In a day when divorce was rare, my father's alcoholic mother was married five times and the stream of men that passed under her roof had little time to invest in his seemingly insignificant life. Naturally, he found his significance among other boys who were also angry and broken. By age sixteen he was in jail and probably on his way to a life of incarceration.

But God intervened in my dad's headlong plunge into delinquency and radically changed the trajectory of his life at a fireside camp service. He made a public profession of faith in Jesus Christ and surrendered to His purposes. Richard had literally walked out of darkness and into the light, and the freedom he experienced propelled him into an unlikely life of ministry that positively impacted thousands of people.

His marriage lasted fifty-five years and produced four children and thirteen grandchildren, all serving Christ. He earned a Doctorate of Ministry and planted two thriving churches. He was leader to a host of grateful parishioners, who credited him with leading them to Christ and discipling them to maturity. This is the wonder, power, and provision of a God who mends broken things and "accomplishes more than we can ask or think," despite ourselves.

But here's the rub that breaks my heart: *He could have accomplished much more.*

My father's profound impact for the Kingdom all but ended when, after an unpleasant and abrupt departure from a church he had founded, his already declining health became the unwelcome constant in a life that had been thrown an unexpected vocational curve. At a time in his life when I know he longed to leverage his wisdom and experience, he became increasingly sidelined—a victim of his life stage. Due to his failing health, he didn't possess the physical and emotional vigor required for reimagining his earthly role in God's Kingdom.

The all-too-common pastoral birthright had been evident for years: a magnetic attraction to stress. Because of this and his family's history of high blood pressure, he took blood pressure medication. He had a deferred prostate condition that led to a series of unsuccessful operations. Finally, a heart attack struck him, leading to subsequent stent and heart bypass procedures. At the time, none of these were imminently life-threatening, but the cumulative and progressive weight took their toll.

A pursuit of healthy eating and fitness was not part of the DNA for most of my father's generation, and he did not look there for answers when he was ill. "Better living through pharmacology" was the prevailing alternative as a long list of prescriptions were enlisted to do battle with a mushrooming log of sympathetic conditions: retinal bleeding, an overactive salivary gland, an undiagnosed and debilitating pain in his stomach, and an understandable battle with depression. Strong pain medication was added to the arsenal. His physical state precluded much fellowship, and my father's calendar was instead filled with doctor appointments and constant fatigue. I'm sure at times my father felt trapped in his own body.

I know my dad loved me and my siblings, loved my mom, loved Jesus, and believed in the work of the church. He had expressed his love to each in tangible and memorable ways over many years. Despite the crumbling foundation he'd inherited, he had given his life to the things of God and had achieved rare success. To God be the glory!

But it seems to me there was unfinished work to be done. I'm confident he felt this as well. With a different perspective on diet, medications, and fitness, I believe my father would have had the physical and emotional strength to invest himself in more profitable and fulfilling late-life endeavors. My family, the local church body, and the community at large would all have benefited from that time and investment.

So as I looked down on my father's face for the last time, I'm filled with not only love, gratitude, and sympathy, but also loss, regret, and emptiness. Memories of care, sacrifice, faithfulness, guidance, and support incongruously joined hands with gnawing questions about what could have been. Had my father been chosen to endure an unwanted gauntlet of sanctification or were lifestyle choices at work here?

My father's life is one of the things that compelled me to embark on this book and the principles it champions. To a degree, he was a product of a generation that includes many who do not emphasize fitness, while maintaining an unblinking trust in the health system. I've lived my life with different priorities and convictions in this area, and I trust that my investments in my health will pay dividends in the years ahead for both my family and the Kingdom of God.

You might think that the state you grew up in or where you currently reside wouldn't make a big impact on your body image or diet and fitness perspective. But in my case, I think they have had at least a moderate influence.

I was a pastor's kid, raised in the Southern California city of Mission Viejo, about halfway between Los Angeles and San Diego. Our coastal neighbors were Newport Beach, Laguna Beach, and San Clemente. In addition to being "the land of fruits and nuts," California is one of a few states (including such places as Colorado and Florida) where people are able to exercise outside nearly year-round. Recreational pursuits are encouraged, and fitness centers are everywhere. People expose plenty of skin, and body consciousness is pretty high. I was no different. I'd frequently appear shirtless at the beach or pool, and this had at least a moderate impact on my thinking.

My spiritual life began as a young boy; responding with childlike faith to the offer of forgiveness God extended to me through Jesus' shed blood on the cross. A simple yet monumental prayer of confession and belief began a journey of trans-formation that continues to this day.

I had two other brothers close in age, and we often participated with neighbor-hood kids in outdoor games and sports that today seem to be part of a bygone era. We spent our afternoons at the pool or beach; playing pick-up games of baseball, whiffle ball, or pickle; and enjoying adventurous hikes or bike rides.

It wasn't until high school, however, that I was consistently involved in any kind of organized athletics beyond a Little League team or a brush with YMCA track and basketball. The summer before my freshman year, a lady in our church cornered me one day and recruited me for her husband's high school wrestling team. Thanks in part to an old set of weights, I possessed a fairly stocky build, and was flattered that someone had seen some athletic potential in me.

Wrestling became one of the most formative experiences of my life. It helped mold my standards of what it means to be fit, healthy, and "in shape," as well as giving me a heightened awareness of the calorie values of various foods.

Our team was very competitive, and if I was to claim a lineup spot I was required to drop weight. At times this became pretty extreme and perhaps unhealthy, as I had to rid myself of nearly all my body fat. My routines included wearing rubber suits (to promote water loss during workouts), taking saunas, missing meals, and running each morning before school. My routines must have seemed crazy to most. I remember my teammates and I chewing a gum high in citric acid to encourage salivation and then spitting into cups on the way to matches. We tried everything we knew to wring out the last ounces necessary to make weight.

Through wrestling, I developed a heightened sense of what it meant to be in top condition. I learned some valuable lessons about weight loss and weight gain that have informed my fitness philosophy ever since. The weekly regimen of making weight for wrestling matches taught me that weight gain and weight loss are a fairly simple formula of calories consumed and calories burned. To lose weight, burn more calories than you consume. To gain weight, consume more calories than you burn. This no-frills, common sense revelation has saved me a lot of confusion and money over the years.

Succeeding as an individual in sports has paid dividends throughout my adult life. While an individual on a team might be able to have his or her mediocre performance overcome by excellent play from teammates, there was no such shelter for me on the wrestling mat or at the pole vault pit. When I'm at the gym today, I notice that people who have the most consistent workout patterns and best results are those that participated in more individualized sports in high school and college.

Sports, especially wrestling, were very challenging and there were many times I wanted to quit. But the satisfaction of reaching personal goals and helping my team kept me going. Deep down I think there was a sense that I was honoring God in what I was doing athletically. People knew I was a professing Christian, and I felt good about giving my best effort as a practical expression of my faith.

While my experiences in athletics were very positive on balance, my involvement in organized athletic endeavors ended in high school. Since that time my life, like yours, has confronted obstacles to a healthy, balanced lifestyle. Some of the obstacles are rooted in habits formed during my youth.

- I have no memory of my parents ever being involved in exercise or fitness programs of any kind.

- My family ate on a tight budget, which meant lots of hamburgers, tuna casseroles, slow-cooker meals, and pot pies.

- There were lots of sugary breakfast cereals, white bread, margarine, store-bought cookies, and heavily sweetened drinks.

- As a child, I began my life-long love affair with candy.

As an adult, I had more stumbling blocks to hurdle, if I was to stay healthy and fit.

- During our four-year yuppie period, Beth and I often ate out at restaurants.

- The culture of my first two jobs (spanning thirteen years) included eating lunch out nearly every day.

- I worked for over eleven years developing a regional ice cream manufacturing and distribution company. Job requirements (I use that term loosely) included taste-testing ice cream, frozen desserts and novelties.

- I spent increasing amounts of time on the road.

- We had a family tradition of big family meals at restaurants after church each Sunday.

- My aging body seemed to hang onto fat more easily as I entered my forties and didn't recover quickly from stress and injury as I entered my fifties.

On the positive side, there have been factors in my life circumstances prodding me and helping me to stay in good shape.

- Because I am a songwriter and musical artist, my picture has been plastered around the community on posters and flyers.

- The pastoral position I have held for many years carries with it an expectation that I am living a life in balance.

- I have a wife who has been supportive of me, interested in maintaining fitness in her own life, and has provided healthy meals for our family.

- I've had access to health care and good information about health.

- I've been able to afford a gym membership.

- I've weaned myself off the only long-term prescription I've ever taken.

But to date, I've never participated in a competitive race over five miles. And I've never had a personal training session or been on any formal diet.

Perhaps you can relate to much of this. Perhaps not. But I suspect most of my life experience may sound familiar to many. We all face fitness and nutrition challenges. Each of our stories is unique, and we all inherit genetics that have the potential to be positive as well as problematic for our health. Additionally, our life experiences and living situations may have supported healthy living or put obstacles in our way. While you might not agree with the conclusions I draw or prescriptions I give, hopefully you can see that my life includes experiences and circumstances similar to those of many others.

CHAPTER 6

JOE'S STORY

Reading a story like David's gives me a deep conviction of God's providence and convinces me that God possesses a sense of humor. That our disparate lives would connect at all, much less lead to a deep and enduring friendship, will remain one of the defining experiences of my life. While David's Southern California upbringing had its rough moments, equating his experiences with mine is like comparing a bumper car ride at the county fair with a thrill ride at Cedar Point, roller coaster capital of the world. While David got jostled a bit within a cocoon of safety (and early faith), most of my life has been a stomach-churning white knuckler.

You may be asking why our stories are relevant for a book about fitness. After all, don't you just need some inspiration, a pat on the fanny, and some sound information on diet and exercise? Apparently not. As has been stated, there are plenty of books covering those topics gathering dust on the bookshelves of an increasingly unhealthy citizenry. What's in short supply are books that tackle the mental, spiritual, and interpersonal battles that occur when we are challenged to think rightly about our bodies. When we pursue a lifestyle of worship—a holistic and biblically-informed balance of mind, body, and spirit with exaltation of God at the center—we are not only running against the grain of our culture, we are becoming spiritually dangerous. You can count on resistance from the world, the flesh, and the Devil (1 John 2:16, Ephesians 6:12). Wrong thinking has typified my life, and I hope that in sharing my experiences you can identify warning signs and find hope and victory over all three of our mutual adversaries.

My story is one of doing everything the world's way—following its script—and, by all outward appearances, finding success. I possessed the superficial marks of health and fitness, while simultaneously unraveling on the inside and in my relationships. Now saved by faith in Jesus, I still battle the temptation to place an unhealthy emphasis on the physical area of life.

People run far, train hard, and sculpt their bodies for a whole host of reasons that have nothing to do with a passion for personal health. Some people run just to get away. Others bulk up to find love and acceptance. Looking back, I trained hard for these reasons as well as to simply survive.

I was born in Clarksburg, West Virginia, in the mid-1960's; the fourth of my parent's five children. Married young, my mom and dad were poorly equipped to handle the stress and expense of raising the Tewell brood. Dad took physically demanding jobs in coal mines and oil fields, while my mom worked sporadically in factories. The love they possessed for their children was most often expressed through providing food, shelter, and clothing, if not intimacy and instruction.

When I was very young our family moved from West Virginia to Oskaloosa, Iowa, where my dad had an opportunity to apply his mining experience to drilling water wells. He was out of town for two to three weeks at a time; my mother worked the second shift at a local factory. Family dinners were rare. I remember hearing my mom's ride home from work entering our driveway at 2 a.m. Mondays, Wednesdays, and Fridays. After I awoke on many Tuesdays, Thursdays, and Saturdays, I would find Mom face-down on the living room couch, still fully clothed and purse over her shoulder. She was sleeping off the previous night's alcohol binge. She was trying to cope the only way she knew how with the reality that she was virtually a single mom. On her off-nights from work, she would stay up late and, before going to her empty bed, crack open my bedroom door to check on me. I remember a small shaft of light from the hallway fanning out across the wall as she peered at me in weary silence. The light dispelled the darkness that surrounded me but retreated all too soon. Darkness seemed to be encroaching on my life as well—a life that should have been carefree, but was becoming increasingly turbulent.

With three older siblings I grew up fast and, without adult supervision or a spiritual compass, I was thrust into situations no child should experience. By the time I was eleven years old, alcohol flowed freely and parties with my friends were common. As a sixth-grader, I routinely came home from school for lunch and ended up using marijuana, instead of having a peanut butter and jelly sandwich and a glass of milk.

As I entered my teens, these "gateway drugs" gave way to uppers, downers, and many others. My buffet of contraband did nothing to satiate my hunger for love, affirmation, and purpose.

Both my grandmothers possessed spiritual life, but our home stayed just out of reach of their invitations to Bible studies, Vacation Bible School, and bedtime prayers. Their influence, though muted, was still profound. Because of their example and moral standards, I was keenly aware that what I was doing was wrong. But at this stage of my life, the Gospel they were living was only an "aroma that leads to death." I knew God's presence marked their lives, but I was unwilling to accept God's love. In part this was because I was a rebel at heart and wanted to live my way. It would also be true to say that I was feeling increasingly unlovable.

I also remember the night my sister was beaten and injured so badly that she was rushed to the hospital. Because I was terrified, confused, anxious, angry, and scared, I was compelled to do something that would both channel and exorcise my despair. For some reason, I reflexively went into the backyard and cracked out one hundred push-ups.

I know that there is no place that is too far from God that His love is not able to go farther still and meet us. My first encounter with His prodigal love came when I was fifteen years old. I was in the throes of the worst drug binge I'd yet pursued. Lying in a vacant campground in Oskaloosa, Iowa, I was paralyzed, numb, empty, despondent, and felt close to death. I wanted all the hurt and pain in my young life to end. Through mingled tears, I told God that if He'd rescue me I would try to be a better person. Even in my drug-addled fog, I think that may have been the first sincere prayer of my life. I wasn't ready to give my life to Jesus yet, but it was becoming clear to me that that I was on a path to nowhere good.

If I had any chance of surviving into adulthood, I needed to find a different circle of friends. Sober people. People with goals. At a pick-up game of football with some other eighth grade boys, a ninth grade football coach approached me about going out for the team the next fall. Never having played with a real team, I was concerned about my abilities, but he assured me I had good hand coordination and natural speed.

A stunned group of faces greeted me at the first practice. There were whispers among the other players, asking, *"Is the drug kid really going out for football?!"* My raggedy gym shorts and torn tennis shoes stood in stark contrast to my well-provisioned teammates. It soon became clear I was an unwelcome intruder in this new world.

When they saw what I could do on the football field, however, everything turned around. Suddenly I had friends—"normal" friends—and I was being given entrée into a place that had previously been unknown to me: a world of relative stability. Here, I was recognized and affirmed by my abilities and contributions, rather than my willingness to join others in mutual debasement.

While I was still a periodic substance abuser, I increasingly traded illicit drugs for more socially acceptable drugs—performance and appearance. I found acceptance among a whole new class of people as my athletic prowess proved invaluable to local baseball and football teams. In addition to the fans in the stands, my female classmates also found me attractive, and the results I was finding in the weight room did nothing but enhance my stature with others.

Against all odds, I secured a scholarship to play football and baseball at Mid-America Nazarene University, in a suburb of Kansas City. This was a strange and promising turn of events as none of my family had attended college, much less a faith-based institution. My mother started attending a church and I was there frequently enough Sundays to compel the pastor to write a letter of recommendation that would pass the sniff test with school trustees. I'd picked up enough Christian jargon from my grandmothers, my mom, and church services to bluff my way through the interview process and found myself on my own for the first time in a big city.

Facing academic rigor for the first time and given freedom to chart my own course without a map to guide me, I reverted to familiar modes of coping. An unholy alliance of recreational drugs and an unbalanced focus on sports left me academically and personally ineligible before the end of my first year. Stung by the realization of the opportunity I'd lost and the embarrassment I'd caused my family, I resolved to land on my feet.

While I didn't possess the academic trappings of success, I still had an ace in the hole: my ability to project a healthy image and positive persona, which others longed to emulate. You can't learn this in a textbook or a college lecture hall. I knew I had it and wanted to leverage it any way possible. Kansas City became my playground, and an outpost of a national fitness center was my personal sandbox.

Amassing the certifications and experience necessary to advance in the fitness industry, it wasn't long before I was managing clubs. I discovered I had an intuitive gift for transforming, within an hour, a cold, club-shopping prospect into an inspired new member with a signed one-year membership agreement. This made me invaluable to the business because signing up people is the mother's milk of chain fitness clubs. The turnover is swift. As one person comes into the system, another departs.

I was expected to produce numbers, not fitness results. I understood that most people walking in the front door were shopping for a new image, not a change of lifestyle. In many ways I represented what they I wanted—a cut, muscular body that exuded energy, confidence, and sex appeal. The implication was that if they joined my club, they could obtain these very things—though the deal didn't guarantee actual health or balance.

I look back with a mixture of amusement and regret at the ways my staff and I cultivated and sustained this goal with current and potential members. I instituted a "pump room," where my staff and I would perform high-repetition exercises with dumbbells just prior to meeting with clients touring our facilities. Emerging from this sales-prep room, I had a ripped look. Like any seasoned salesman, I knew what phrases, compliments, challenges, and expiring-today sales pitches to present and when to offer them. For the Christians that sat at my desk, I understood enough of their dialect to give every indication that I, too, was a brother in the faith. But as with so many other products, I wasn't selling reality so much as I was selling an image and a dream.

The truth is, the image I was projecting was made possible only with the aid of products not legally available to my clients. While I'd spent years chiseling my body to near perfection, the results I was obtaining were not possible without the use of anabolic steroids—drugs I'd deemed necessary to maintain my credibility as a top fitness coach. The confidence and personal interest I exuded were covers for my shaky self-esteem, drug-fueled stamina, and an incessant need to impress every attractive female in my sight.

My senses went on high alert the night a fit, blonde socialite with magazine beauty approached me for a personal training package. I cleared my schedule and soon fell under the spell of this high-bred, intelligent, ambitious woman. She possessed everything I thought I wanted: beauty, competence, a stable family, a drive to succeed, and an unspoken understanding that image is everything.

But after a few years together, I discovered that it takes more than mutual ambition and well-polished images to make a relationship work. At the time, it seemed like I had life by the tail. But looking back, I can see it was all a tragic façade.

The sad truth is I was pushing my body beyond what it was made to withstand, both physically and chemically. An invasive surgery to repair my neck and recurring irritation in my shoulders are daily reminders of my former excess. I had successfully escaped the youthful prison of socially unacceptable addictions and habits only to trade them for new, more acceptable forms of incarceration.

I made my living by coaching people toward my version of a better life—a stronger and more resilient mind and body—even as I poisoned my own. The realization that life wasn't working out for me was running in ironic tandem with my job. Clients came to me daily with the expectation I would infuse passion into them so they could achieve my kind of successful life. The dissonance between this premise and reality of my so-called success was making me very angry. Rather than dealing with the source of my problems, I threw myself into a partnership at a new club in a Des Moines suburb. I pursued relationships and aggressively lifted weights. I had to keep moving forward—*I couldn't fail.* Failure was for people like the family I'd left behind in Oskaloosa.

The mess my life was becoming had not gone unnoticed by my business partner.

FIT FOR THE KING

He was concerned not only for me personally, but for the toll my choices were going to take on our business. His moral perspective was becoming clearer thanks to a believing wife and a recent decision to follow Jesus. When he had proof I was involved with a current member of our club, he called in reinforcements.

Answering the call was David Bush (my good friend and co-author of this book), a local Christian musician and worship leader. David and his wife were regulars at our fitness club and had talked with my partner about their mutual relationship with Christ. I'll never forget the afternoon David showed up unexpectedly at the gym and asked if I'd take a walk with him around the nearby lake. I tried to blow him off, but my partner insisted this was an appointment I had to take.

Leaving the building under duress, I had a premonition that some kind of hammer was about to fall. I'd had the same uncomfortable feeling several weeks earlier when I was at David and Beth's home for a dinner party. In contrast to what I saw in their lives and experienced with them, I felt deep conviction regarding my duplicitous lifestyle. I felt for most of the evening that I was either going to bolt from the house or fall on my face and confess everything right then and there.

David's first question hit me right between the eyes: "Joe, why are you so angry and bitter?"

There it was. *The big question* nobody had ever asked, probably because nobody would believe that a guy with my trappings of success could be anything but happy, secure, and self-sufficient. *Did he know the dirty little secret of people like me?* I wondered. *Could he possibly know that my pursuits of performance, perfection, control, recognition, achievement, and women fed off of resentment and a constant need to prove my worth?*

I was disarmed and we began a conversation that changed my life. Through David's questions, sincere concern, and statements of biblical truth, the Holy Spirit exposed the sin in my life. For some reason, I didn't want to run anymore. I had a deep desire to be freed from all my compulsions, lies, and hypocrisy. Before long, I found myself calling out to God again, like I had so many years before in the abandoned campground in Oskaloosa. Only this time, I didn't want to simply be spared the consequences of my stupidity and rebellion. There was deep remorse over how I ignored and offended my Creator and the legacy of pain and dysfunction I was perpetuating.

Tears streaked my face that day—tears that poured from a heart and a life that was broken. I was done pretending that life on my terms worked. I asked Jesus for forgiveness, and He gave to me what He alone can give. I literally felt a weight lifted from me. I didn't know what all this would mean going forward, but I left a lakeside park bench that day feeling more peace, freedom, and acceptance from God than I'd ever experienced. I wasn't alone, running away from a troubled past and disdainful pedigree. I was His child now. Jesus was with me.

I would love to tell you that everything changed for me that day, but it didn't. Praise God, my sins were forgiven, my eternal destiny changed, and I had a new moral compass courtesy of the Holy Spirit. The trajectory of my life was transformed, but I was still clearly a work in progress. I had to clean up the mess I'd been making of my life, including the habits and behaviors that had become instinctual and my reflexive ways of coping with stress and disappointment. These aspects of my character were now headwinds I would face as I learned to tack for calmer waters with the help of the Holy Spirit and the body of Christ.

In many ways I've also had to re-evaluate my motivations for pursuing fitness and helping others develop fit lifestyles. The things that had previously fueled my fire—success, notoriety, vanity, and self-worth—were still in play, but were increasingly replaced by more foundational and worthy motivations. Learning and developing the principles presented in this book have been instructive for my life, and I've experienced more joy and satisfaction in a balanced pursuit of holistic fitness for the right reasons than I ever did as a high-octane fitness junkie.

Do our personal stories matter? Is a fit lifestyle more than a club membership? Is it possible that our current thinking about fitness, our bodies, and our intrinsic value needs to be destroyed so a proper foundation can be laid? I believe the answer to these questions is an emphatic "Yes!" Our culture is not providing us with honest answers or appropriate motivation for physical and spiritual transformation. Embrace the destruction of your flawed thinking. Courageously begin to lay a new foundation. Dare to believe in a better life animated by God's unconditional love. With God's help I have, and I'm a better man for it.

PART THREE
DEMOLITION

CHAPTER 7

JESUS LOVES ME, THIS I ... ?

Growing up, I'd been given the unenviable designation of being "Overdo Dave." My father appropriately gave this title to me, as even today I find myself tempering an inner drive to do things in complex, unique, or extravagant ways. Good things can and have come from this tendency in my adult years, but as an adolescent and young adult there were not many positive ways to express my natural bias. I know I frustrated my dad with clubhouses that consumed all his tools and spare plywood, school projects that ended up drawing upon limited resources, social activities that started too early and ended too late, high school wrestling diet and workout regimens that were over the top, and photo shoots and publicity pieces that were beyond the pale. Through my teenage years, dad would often end up holding the bag somehow to either execute my ideas or salvage them. While I didn't really appreciate hearing "there goes overdo Dave again," I can understand now as a father of four how exasperating some of my escapades must have been.

Having not learned my lesson yet, I set out as a nineteen-year-old to produce a benefit concert for my school district's music departments in a local auditorium. I had given many well-attended concerts in the past, and trusted this one would be no different. I was so confident that I hired in lights, sound, an all-star back-up band, and printed programs. I was on the hook for close to $2000—and that was real money back in 1982.

The night of the concert my hometown experienced a rare deluge of rain and attendance was not near what I had expected or needed. In the afterglow came the unsettling reality that after my own resources were tapped, I was still short over $1000 needed to pay the bills. My dad knew I had taken a bath on the event and the next night he called me into his home office.

Like the prodigal son returning from a distant land, I prepared myself for the justifiable lecture I would receive. *You're an adult now, when are you going to start acting like one? How long am I going to have to keep paying for your boondoggles? I knew this was not going to end well. Why couldn't you see it? What is it going to take to stop being "Overdo Dave"?*

Dad would have been right. I deserved whatever he was going to dish out. *When was I ever going to learn? I was such a failure.*

But that's not what happened.

After I confessed how much I owed and to whom, he calmly got out his checkbook and started writing checks—paying every debt in full. Then he did something even more unexpected ... something I'll never forget. He got up from his desk and hugged me. He told me he loved me. He said he was certain I would grow up to be a good man and a great husband.

What was this!? The checks were enough to cover the debt I couldn't pay. Was dad also choosing to overlook and forgive my obvious shortcomings? Amidst my character flaws—flaws that continued to carry a price tag for him—did he believe something about me that I wasn't sure I even believed myself?

Experiencing God's Unconditional Love

It's a wonderful thing to be surprised by grace. More wonderful still when we can accept and own it. Because we are "in Christ," we have been found worthy of receiving grace. This is the clear message of Scripture; but many aren't buying it. Tripped up by worldly definitions of love, many refuse to believe the foundational revelation that *God Is Love* and *God Loves Us (1 John 4:10; John 3:16).*

Somewhere in the back of our minds is the certainty that we are constantly disappointing God. But to be disappointed with us, God would have to be surprised by our conduct—expecting a different or better result than what He got. Because God is not surprised by anything we do, this is not an option (Ps 139:15-16). The Apostle Paul makes it clear in Ephesians that God chose us for a special love relationship with Him in spite of all the shortcomings we bring to the table.

> *Even before He made the world, God loved us and chose us in Christ to be holy and without fault in His eyes. God decided in advance to adopt us into His own family by bringing us to Himself through Jesus Christ. This is what He wanted to do, and it gave Him great pleasure. Ephesians 1:4-5 (NLT)*

God doesn't love us more or less depending on our ability to perform to His standards. He doesn't lower the standards, but His love is not constrained by this because *in Christ* we have perfectly met His standards. He loves us because He loves Jesus and sees Him in us, because we're made in His image, and because He's chosen to do so. It's that incomprehensible, yet that simple.

When our repeated failures and shortcomings seem to be constantly on parade, it's no wonder so many construct elaborate defenses against God's grace and love. Where such defenses exist, these emotional fortresses can't help but morph into the physical arena of our lives, manifesting themselves as performance-driven acceptance, body-image issues, and self-loathing. ***These powerful, negative and misguided perceptions of our value must be demolished before a secure foundational perspective of diet and fitness can be built.*** Until this rubble is cleared away, we are not thinking biblically and our efforts to develop new patterns of thinking and living will be sabotaged.

The Pocket Full of Rocks band expresses well God's unconditional love.

Come As You Are

He's not mad at you
And He's not disappointed
His grace is greater still
Than all of your wrong choices

He is full of mercy
And He is ever kind
Hear His invitation
His arms are open wide

You can come as you are with all your broken pieces
And all your shameful scars
The pain you hold in your heart, bring it all to Jesus
You can come as you are

Louder than the voice
That whispers you're unworthy
Hear the sound of love
That tells a different story

Shattering your darkness
And pushing through the lies
How tenderly He calls you
His arms are open wide

You can come as you are with all your broken pieces
And all your shameful scars
The pain you hold in your heart, you bring it all to Jesus
You can come as you are

Words by Michael Farren, Chad Cates and Tony Wood
©2009 Pocket Full Of Rocks Publishing/Word Music/Cates By Cates
Music/Sony/ATV Cross Keys Publishing/Songs From Exit 71
Used by permission

Who We Are In Christ

Far too often, our journey toward sustainable fitness is detoured not because our bodies won't cooperate, but because we haven't settled in our minds who we are in Christ. The security and perfection of His love tempers the performance addicts who never sense they've arrived, as well as the easily defeated individual whose low sense of self-worth keeps him or her on the sidelines.

In a very real sense, our bodies are a visible testimony to the value we perceive we have in the eyes of God. It seems apparent that many people do not understand or have not fully accepted the love that God has for them. The Apostle Paul reminds us of the critical need to think rightly and not let our flesh or our culture sow seeds of doubt on issues to which the Bible speaks clearly.

> *We are destroying speculations and every lofty thing raised up against the knowledge of God, and we are taking every thought captive to the obedience of Christ. 2 Corinthians 10:5 (NASB)*

One of the most basic and glorious truths we are taught from an early age is that God is Love, and His love is personally bestowed upon us. His love is experienced by all people everywhere through His common graces: sun, rain, beauty, our senses, music, capabilities, children, delicious food, interpersonal love, and a host of other manifestations. These are all His ideas and they are accessible to everyone regardless of their acknowledgement of Him. He simply chooses to give them.

Those who are in a relationship with Jesus obtain an incomprehensively greater number of blessings because of their union with Him.

> *All praise to God, the Father of our Lord Jesus Christ, who has blessed us with every spiritual blessing in the heavenly realms because we are united with Christ … so we praise God for the glorious grace He has poured out on us who belong to His dear Son. Ephesians 1:3, 6 (NLT)*

"Every spiritual blessing" includes the sealing presence, gifts, and leading of His Holy Spirit; our ability to understand Scripture; our desire to obey Him; the inheritance we will enjoy with Him in Heaven; and many other things. With all this love coming our way from no less than the Creator of the universe, how is it possible that so many feel unloved or unlovable? Somewhere between the child-like acceptance of our worth through the eyes of a loving God and our transition into adolescence, we begin to question our worthiness as objects of God's love and grace. (Many do not struggle with self-worth but do tend to place an unhealthy emphasis on the physical and superficial aspects of their lives. More on this in Chapter 8.) *It's quite possible that when we don't follow His best for our lives in the physical arena, we begin a downward spiral of doubt, wrong thinking, and subsequent behavior that metastasizes, affecting our self-image and sense of worth.* Repenting, right thinking, and obedience can reverse this debilitating spiral in our physical bodies just as it does in the rest of our lives.

God's Unique Love

Because most of the love we experience from other people is conditional, it is hard for us to think and operate under God's umbrella of *unconditional* love. While we may aspire to demonstrate unconditional love to others, the reality is that our fallen human nature makes this a rarer occurrence than we'd care to admit (Romans 7:21-22). Stop performing and responding the way your friends and family expect, and before long you can expect to feel the cold embrace of *conditional love.* In the first flush of infatuated love, some might express the sentiments of this Billy Joel song:

Just The Way You Are

Don't go changing, to try and please me
You never let me down before
Don't imagine you're too familiar
And I don't see you anymore

I would not leave you in times of trouble
We never could have come this far
I took the good times, I'll take the bad times
I'll take you just the way you are

Words and Music by Billy Joel © 1977 and 1978 Impulsive Music

But after a litany of letdowns, the tediousness of the familiar, and more bad times than good, it's safe to assume even Billy would be asking for a do-over. All romantic smarminess aside, most people are more familiar with this popular Carole King song as the soundtrack to their closest relationships:

It's Too Late

It used to be so easy living here with you
You were light and breezy and I knew just what to do

Now you look so unhappy, and I feel like a fool
And it's too late, baby, now it's too late
Though we really did try to make it
Something inside has died and I can't hide
And I just can't fake it

There'll be good times again for me and you
But we just can't stay together, don't you feel it too
Still I'm glad for what we had, and how I once loved you

But it's too late, baby, it's too late
Though we really did try to make it
Something inside has died and I can't hide
And I just can't fake it

Words and Music by Carole King and Toni Stern
©1971 (Renewed 1999) Colgems-EMI Music
Used by permission

It should be a comforting truth to know that God will never be singing that over our lives! He is not surprised by our shortcomings, so He's not disappointed with us. He sees our lives as being in Christ, and because Christ perfectly pleases Him, we are pleasing to Him as well (Colossians 1:19-22).

The fact that God is not disappointed with us does not mean that He doesn't *disapprove* of some of our thoughts and actions. God clearly sees things in our lives as regrettable, fruitless, dishonoring, and shameful. But His justifiable perspective does not cause Him to be disappointed in us or to love us any less than He ever has.

Breaking the Bondage of Performance

The reason we can be so confident in the stability and unconditional nature of God's love is because we did nothing to cause Him to love us in the first place. Before we existed, He chose to love us for His own purposes and glory—not as a response to something admirable He saw us doing somewhere down the corridors of time. The Prophet Isaiah shares with us God's perspective of our attempts to please Him via good performance.

We are all infected and impure with sin. When we display our righteous deeds, they are nothing but filthy rags. Like autumn leaves, we wither and fall, and our sins sweep us away like the wind.
Isaiah 64:6 (NLT)(Emphasis mine)

The people of Israel are a prime example of the uncaused nature of God's love. He chose to bless and use the Israelites not because of their size, stature, obedience, philanthropy, or inclination to love Him.

"For you are a holy people, who belong to the LORD your God. Of all the people on earth, the LORD your God has chosen you to be his own special treasure. The LORD did not set his heart on you and choose you because you were more numerous than other nations, for you were the smallest of all nations! Rather, it was simply that the LORD loves you, and he was keeping the oath he had sworn to your ancestors. That is why the LORD rescued you with such a strong hand from your slavery and from the oppressive hand of Pharaoh, king of Egypt." Deuteronomy 7:6-8 (NLT)

God's love is divorced from performance. He graciously extended his unconditional love to us when we were in direct opposition to Him.

But God showed his great love for us by sending Christ to die for us while we were still sinners. Romans 5:8 (NLT)

Believing and Accepting God's Love

What is standing between you and the full acceptance of God's love? Why don't you receive as a gift the acceptance and ownership of God that puts to rest the lies, opinions, doubts, and self-fulfilling prophecies of failure you've repeatedly experienced in the area of body care? *Identifying, repenting, and speaking the truth into these deceptions and distortions is a critical first step toward becoming* **Fit For The King.** Review the Scripture that's been shared in this chapter. Memorize it, personalize it, and internalize it. May God's words of love and affirmation overwhelm other voices that may be proclaiming a false message regarding your value, worthiness, or capacity to be loved.

It's altogether possible you are learning for the first time about the kind of love God has for His children. You may feel as though you're eavesdropping on a family conversation you're not sure you're a part of. You believe that

57

you've been a recipient of many of the common graces of a loving God, but you do not experience the kind of intimacy that is described in the Bible:

And because we are his children, God has sent the Spirit of his Son into our hearts, prompting us to call out, "Abba [Daddy], Father." Now you are no longer a slave but God's own child. And since you are his child, God has made you his heir. Galatians 4:6-7 (NLT)

The special love God has for His children is entirely due to the fact that they have become related to Him through Jesus. When a person accepts God's gift of Jesus, they not only experience a fresh revelation of the depths of His unique love, they also personally experience God's *forgiveness*. Everyone is an object of God's love, and all experience many manifestations of it each day. God's special grace, mercy, and forgiveness, however, are the gifts He gives to those who place their faith in Jesus—God's only provision for reconciling our estranged relationship with Him.

You've purchased this book because you're interested in gaining a biblical perspective on health and fitness. While I obviously believe the Bible has a lot to say on this topic, the overarching message of the Bible is that God's ultimate expression of love for us was providing Jesus as the solution to our universal problem of sin, which separates us from experiencing the fullness of His love. This chapter begins the work of demolishing wrong thinking about our worthiness and identity that leads to wrong actions. As long as we're demolishing lies and fallacies that condemn us to failure in our efforts to change physically, we might as well take a wrecking ball to these other falsehoods we often believe about ourselves:

- We're basically good people
- God helps those who help themselves
- The good things in our lives will ultimately outweigh the bad
- Because God loves us, our eternal future is secure

Your vigorous pursuit of fitness may be your way of proving one or more of the statements above. Perhaps your belief in these things allows you to comfortably exist in a poor state of health.

Whatever the case, here's the reality God paints for us:

There is none righteous, not even one. Romans 3:10 (NASB)

For all have sinned and fall short of the glory of God. Romans 3:23 (NASB)

For the wages of sin is death, but the free gift of God is eternal life through Christ Jesus our Lord. Romans 6:23 (NLT)

Jesus told him, "I am the way, the truth, and the life. No one can come to the Father except through me." John 14:6 (NLT)

God saved you by his grace when you believed. And you can't take credit for this; it is a gift from God. Salvation is not a reward for the good things we have done, so none of us can boast about it. Ephesians 2:8-9 (NLT)

As important as it is for us to demolish wrong thinking about our worth and dignity, I would strongly encourage you to evaluate where you stand with Jesus. Becoming physically fit does not require a relationship with Jesus, but being spiritually fit for an intimate and eternal relationship with God most certainly does.

I began this chapter with the story about my father and my failed benefit concert, and you'll remember that in addition to blessing me with words of affirmation, he also paid my substantial debt. As wonderful as his words were, I still would have been financially busted if he hadn't intervened and dealt with a problem he alone had the resources to handle.

A spiritually fit person agrees with God that he or she doesn't meet His standard of perfection. Instead, this person exchanges his or her imperfection for the perfection God offers through His Son Jesus Christ. Are you convicted today that you stand guilty before God and have not received the special love and forgiveness that comes only through Jesus? If so, I would encourage you to talk to God right now about your need for Him and your willingness to receive His precious gift.

Resting in God's Love

In Jesus, God has provided the remedy for our rebellion and the solution to our striving to perform better. He's covered our innate sense of unworthiness through the abundant and perfect worthiness of Christ. He asks us to, by faith, rest in Jesus' accomplishments. Rather than simply trading one kind of taskmaster for another, a life of following Jesus brings with it a whole new way of dealing with the inevitable trials and challenges common to humanity.

"Come to me, all of you who are weary and carry heavy burdens, and I will give you rest. Take my yoke upon you. Let me teach you, because I

am humble and gentle at heart, and you will find rest for your souls. For
my yoke is easy to bear, and the burden I give you is light."
Matthew 11:28-30 (NLT)

As you continue through this book, you will be presented with many practical ways you can take action to become *Fit For The King*. These will be steps of obedience and life stewardship that will produce a life-giving cycle of improved body function and appearance. You will experience many physical and spiritual benefits as a result of these steps. But making progress toward a lifestyle of fitness will not change a thing about God's love for you. His love for you was a settled issue from before the world began. It delights Him to give His unique love and forgiveness to you. All He asks is that you rest in Him.

Jesus I Am Resting, Resting

Jesus I am resting, resting
In the Joy of what Thou art;
I am finding out the greatness
Of Thy loving heart.
Thou hast bid me gaze upon Thee,
And Thy beauty fills my soul,
For by Thy transforming power
Thou hast made me whole.

Simply trusting Thee, Lord Jesus,
I behold Thee as Thou art,
And Thy love, so pure, so changeless,
Satisfies my heart;
Satisfies its deepest longings,
Meets supplies its every need,
Compasseth me round with blessings;
Thine is love indeed!

Jean Pigott and James Mountain. Public Domain

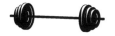

CHAPTER 8
MYTHBUSTERS

So far David has been doing most of the talking, and that's OK. Unless you understand and own the deeper spiritual issues you may have with your body, you won't be looking to me for practical advice and direction. But as you make a commitment to think, live, and act differently, there will be no shortage of obstacles to progress presenting themselves. It would be unrealistic to think that this is your first time to the lifestyle-reboot rodeo. Real or imagined, you have barriers to change that you will need to face.

Following Jesus can be dangerous and requires courage. During Jesus' time of ministry here on earth, there was always a crowd as long as He kept providing food. But when he faced people with the fact that they pursued Him with wrong and self-serving motives, they scattered like cockroaches when the lights come on (John 6:22-27). As the challenges of being a Christ follower arise, I hope you can resist the natural temptation to either rationalize why you are doing this or simply head for the nearest exit.

I'd like to deal with some of the most common reasons I'm given for not pursuing a healthy and balanced lifestyle. I've sat across the desk from literally thousands of deconditioned people over the past twenty-five years and I've probably heard everything when it comes to excuses. A few are legit. Most are smoke screens, and many people have an uncanny ability to lie to themselves. Jesus said that "the truth shall set you free," and in the interest of freedom, I'm going to lay some heavy truth on you in this chapter. Unlike Jack Nicholson's courtroom audience in *A Few Good Men*, hopefully you can handle the truth. Here are ten excuses I've heard repeatedly over the years from people who struggle as they face the truth about their physical condition.

----

1. I can't afford a membership to the gym.

Getting healthy and finding balance in our physical lives doesn't demand a gym membership. In my experience, however, it is an invaluable tool to help you reach your goals. Our culture will continue to make too much food available to the vast majority of people, and our jobs and routines don't usually provide a means for burning off what we're consuming, much less build up muscle density. The average American spends $7 a day on incidentals that lead to health problems—far more than what any gym membership would cost. At a health club you find more than equipment; you find people who can answer questions, people who can encourage you, and people who are not followers of Jesus who need to meet people who know Him. What is more important than your health? Certainly this is worth an investment. If finances are really that tight, try approaching your employer to see if the company will share or even cover the cost of a membership. If that isn't possible, approach a few health clubs and see if you could barter or trade services for a membership. I know a guy who watches the front desk for an hour or so in the early morning (when no one wants to go to work) in trade for a free family membership. With this kind of arrangement, you're even freed from an excuse for why you couldn't make it into the gym!

2. I don't have the time to take care of myself.

We all know that we make time for what's important to us. A significant purpose of this book is to make your health and fitness a balanced priority in your life. Many people "don't have time" to exercise until they have a health scare. Suddenly, they "make time." **For most people, their health problems are a result of what they're eating, not how much exercise they're getting.** Eating less doesn't involve extra time—in fact, it might create extra time. With the right attitude and direction, thirty to forty-five minutes of exercise five days a week is sufficient for most people. One less TV show, a little less Facebook, getting to bed thirty minutes earlier, and planning your day will likely provide most people more than enough time for the gym. When clients insist they don't have time to invest in fitness, they'll often hear me say, "Ignore your health … it'll go away," or another favorite, "If you don't make time to be healthy, you'd better plan to spend time with illness."

3. Exercising in public is embarrassing; I'm not in good shape.

What's more embarrassing: being seen in the gym starting on an exercise routine that will transform your life or being silently judged while you stand in line at a fast-food restaurant? If you've been inside a gym recently, you'll know that it is not just a place for muscle heads to pump iron. Times have changed, and people are used to seeing obese and uninitiated people in a gym. The vast majority of the people who book training sessions with me are badly deconditioned people, not athletes in training.

4. I can do it on my own.

A quote from Dr. Phil is appropriate here: "How's that working for you?" Maybe you *can* do it on your own—*but you haven't*. Joining a club is a statement of intent and lifestyle. If a barrier to joining a health club is present, the chances of making the first steps are usually put off for "another time." Too many people visit hospital rehab units under doctors' orders instead of joining fitness clubs under their own free will. At least at the start of most exercise classes, there are people who will hold you accountable. The other people in the group will help you reach your goals. Programs like Weight Watchers, Rick Warren's Daniel Plan and others are successful largely because of accountability.

5. My body is different than everybody else's.

Every body is not the same, and the goal of this book is not to create some kind of monolithic standard of what everyone should look like. "Fit" people look different, have different dress or pant sizes, and even varying amounts of body fat. Your body is more damaged by your behaviors than by your genetics. With rare exceptions (and most of those are temporary), your weight gain or weight loss is a function of energy in and energy out. To lose weight, you don't need a genetic makeover, you simply need to burn more calories than you're consuming over a protracted period of time. Resistance training builds muscle, a sedentary lifestyle causes atrophy. Stretching increases flexibility, inactivity decreases flexibility. Muscle movement and an increased heart rate burns calories faster than sitting or standing. I'm not book-smart like David—but this makes sense even to me.

6. I can correct my issues through drugs and surgery.

With the amazing advances in science and medicine, it is possible for drugs and surgery to mitigate or postpone the consequences of many of our health issues. For those with high cholesterol, there are statin drugs. For those with high blood pressure, joint pain caused by inflammation, diabetes, sleeplessness, etc., there will always be someone happy to write you prescriptions. For those who feel desperate enough, there's bariatric (weight loss) surgery.

Since when has the knee-jerk reaction of a disciple of Jesus been to get surgery or a drug to deal with an issue? Medicine is a blessing for many people with no other alternative, but it seems that we should determine first if there are indeed "no other alternatives." Changes to our diet and exercise habits provide an option to many of the prescriptions being written today. Most drugs have side effects that can create other, unrelated problems. While drugs or surgery may address the immediate issue that threatens your health, most do nothing to actually make your body healthier, stronger, more resistant to disease and more energetic. Diet and exercise deal with pesky issues like these.

7. Getting in shape is easy and pain-free.

It isn't, regardless of what that commercial for a weight-loss pill just claimed. A heart bypass and life as a diabetic isn't easy, either. Nothing that takes self-control is "easy." Raising good kids isn't easy. Pregnancy and giving birth aren't easy. Keeping a good reputation isn't easy. Honesty isn't easy, and neither is marriage. Managing your money wisely and saving for retirement isn't easy. Following Christ isn't easy. Most good and beneficial things are not easy, but we do them because we know by experience that the reward is worth the temporary pain or inconvenience. Since we don't have the strength to do these hard things, we invite Jesus into the picture on a daily basis because He specializes in making hard and impossible things possible. In contrast, sloth and gluttony are easy. Sitting and resting are easy. Procrastinating, lying, and gossiping are easy. We don't need any help with these things.

8. I just need to find a diet that will work for me.

The great news is that God has already found a great diet for you—it's called fresh, nutritious food. This is different than the food that often comes frozen or shelf stable, has an expiration date of twelve months, includes more than a few ingredients, or only needs you to add water to consume. Real, honest-to-goodness food is usually found in the perimeter areas of your grocery store, as well as at your local farmer's market. At these places, you can buy lean meat, vegetables, fruits, seeds, dairy products, whole grains, and other God-designed foods. Fill your grocery carts, pantries, and refrigerators with these kinds of food. Diets by design are not sustainable, and have done little to change the incremental health problems our nation is facing. To borrow from the myth I busted above, diets are "easy" shortcuts that do not address the fundamental issue of making consistent, wise decisions about what we're going to put in the bodies God has given us. These decisions have become "hard" in the past few decades. We've been lured away from whole foods because prepared foods provide higher profits for food marketers. Food manufacturers are not evil—they are simply meeting a growing demand for quicker, sweeter, nonperishable, and cheaper food. We have growing access to better choices, however, as more people are "going back" to real, fresh food.

In my twenty-five years of experience as a gym owner and trainer, I have seen very few people make significant progress toward losing weight by only following a diet. Nearly everyone will need to change their activity level in coordination with food intake changes. So even if you want to follow a marketed diet program, it's essential that you address the exercise part of the equation, as well.

9. The scale will be my barometer of health.

Scales are good for one thing: telling you what you weigh. They are not good indicators of overall health or fitness. Your clothes and your mobility will tell you as much about the appropriateness of your body size as anything else. Our hospitals and hospices are filled with people who are sick, diseased, and dying who would have confidence that they are in good health based on what they weigh.

10. I struggle losing weight because I have low metabolism.

While there are a few people who have legitimate hormonal issues that affect their metabolism, this is actually quite rare. The main influences on your metabolism are your age, your sex, and your muscle mass. Your metabolism (how quickly you burn calories) slows about 5 percent per decade after age forty, making age an issue for anyone who doesn't adjust his or her consumption while growing older. Men burn calories faster than women, giving them an edge in the metabolism race. The greatest factor, however, is muscle mass, which is why building lean muscle is a critical part of any weight-loss plan. This is also a reason why depending on a diet or reduction in food intake for weight loss is such a long, hard road. The fact is that heavier people have *higher* metabolism than thinner individuals, since their bodies have to work harder to get through each day. This is one major reason heavier people can enjoy rapid weight loss at the beginning of any program. Their higher metabolism is actually working for them. The more weight they lose, the less of a tailwind they have from their metabolic rate.

CHAPTER 9
EDIFICE COMPLEX

Susan Boyle shocked the world at her 2009 audition for *Britain's Got Talent,* when the matronly forty-seven-year-old Brit sang "I Dreamed a Dream" before a gape-mouthed audience. What most viewers assumed would be a performance designed for laughs became a metaphor: Don't judge a person's capacity for greatness by their appearance.

Susan's beautiful singing voice has since afforded her the opportunity to perform and record extensively, resulting in a financial windfall in the millions of pounds. In 2010, she completed construction of a new home—large by British standards— that has become a metaphor of its own. Shaped by a lifetime of frugality, Susan placed restraints on her monthly income to the point that she could not afford to furnish or live in the home, despite her swelling bank account. [1] Impressive from the outside, Ms. Boyle's home was a glorious shell.

Ms. Boyle's story illustrates two corresponding truths that have major implications for followers of Jesus who seek balance in their physical and spiritual lives. First, it's a comforting reality that God is not impressed by appearances. Second, it's relatively easy to impress others with facades that hide spiritual decay, though God is not fooled. While it's easier for Christians to put up fronts than to cultivate spiritual depth, maintaining the bodies we were given should be an outgrowth of biblical conviction rather than an ongoing effort to perpetuate an image.

Keeping Up Appearances

While the average person may have difficulty relating to Susan's rise from anonymity to stardom, many can understand what it means to be "house poor." This is a term that has entered our popular vernacular as homeowners, eager to impress others, purchase more home than they can afford to furnish or adequately repair. While ultra-low teaser interest rates and a desire to "keep up with the Joneses" have fueled an edifice complex in many of our neighborhoods, it's also true that many who fill the pews on Sunday are "house poor" in a different fashion. Physically impressive and well coiffured, no one would suspect that there is spiritual neglect festering just below the surface.

While this book will skew toward readers seeking a healthier future, I am compelled to speak with equal passion to those who have invested heavily in their physical health and appearance to the detriment of their spiritual lives. A biblically-informed balance is the goal, and physical fitness must never be used as cover for spiritual atrophy.

In the Old Testament, the selection of a king for Israel became a costly exercise in learning to see how God sees. Saul, Israel's first king, found favor in the people's eyes because of his impressive physical appearance.

> *[Kish] had a son whose name was Saul, a choice and handsome man, and there was not a more handsome person than he among the sons of Israel; from his shoulders and up he was taller than any of the people.*
> *1 Samuel 9:2 (NASB)*

But Saul's spiritual intransigence eventually disqualified him from leadership.

> *"I [God] regret that I have made Saul king, for he has turned back from following Me and has not carried out My commands." And Samuel was distressed and cried out to the LORD all night. 1 Samuel 15:11 (NASB)*

God's man was David, who had balanced his physical prowess with a heart that was animated by bringing glory and honor to his Creator. But first God had to move the Prophet Samuel beyond his Boylesque judging-by-the-cover prejudices when the oldest of David's brothers presented themselves for consideration as heirs to Saul's throne.

> *When they entered, he [Samuel] looked at Eliab [David's oldest brother] and thought, "Surely the LORD'S anointed is before Him." But the LORD said to Samuel, "Do not look at his appearance or at the height of his stature, because I have rejected him; for God sees not as man sees, for man looks at the outward appearance, but the LORD looks at the heart."*
> *1 Samuel 16:6-7 (NASB)*

In the New Testament, Jesus was adamant about how unimpressed God was with outward appearances that masked spiritual lethargy and lawlessness.

> *"Woe to you, scribes and Pharisees, hypocrites! For you are like white-washed tombs which on the outside appear beautiful, but inside they are*

full of dead men's bones and all uncleanness. So you, too, outwardly
appear righteous to men, but inwardly you are full of hypocrisy
and lawlessness." Matthew 23:27-28 (NASB)

The Apostle Paul concedes that our earthen vessels are decaying but that God can still be glorified in us as we experience daily spiritual renewal through intimacy with Christ.

But we have this treasure in earthen vessels, so that the surpassing great-
ness of the power may be of God and not from ourselves ... therefore
we do not lose heart, but though our outer man is decaying, yet our inner
man is being renewed day by day ... we look not at the things which are
seen, but at the things which are not seen; for the things which are seen
are temporal, but the things which are not seen are eternal.
2 Corinthians 4:7,16,18 (NASB)

We aren't out to impress people with a good image, but to appropriately reflect the image of Christ. While we may be able to fool others into thinking we are spiritually healthy because of our physical appearance, the One who sees through to our hearts is not deceived. Our bodies conform to a high standard of fitness as an appropriate response to the changes Jesus has made in our lives.

Paul reminds us that our motives will be revealed one day:

Anyone who builds on that foundation may use a variety of materials—
gold, silver, jewels, wood, hay, or straw. But on the judgment day, fire
will reveal what kind of work each builder has done. The fire will show if
a person's work has any value. If the work survives, that builder will re-
ceive a reward. But if the work is burned up, the builder will suffer great
loss. The builder will be saved, but like someone barely escaping through
a wall of flames. Don't you realize that all of you together are the temple
of God and that the Spirit of God lives in you?
God will destroy anyone who destroys this temple.
For God's temple is holy, and you are that temple.
1 Corinthians 3:12-16 (NLT)

After a foundation for our faith has been laid on the true Gospel of grace, further construction is to be done with worthy materials. God is pleased with our investments in physical fitness when they are balanced with a passion to know and follow Him as a first priority.

Rethinking Our Priorities

An Old Testament example of this kind of balance is found in the construction and filling of the original Temple in Jerusalem. God enabled a glorious Temple to be built by Solomon to honor His name. It included a "Most Holy Place," the Holy of Holies, where God's presence actually dwelled. 1 Kings chapters 5 and 6 give us the unimaginable scope of its beauty and splendor. God takes up residence in the Temple's inner room between two pure gold cherubim atop the Ark of the Covenant. God dwelling among men! This was unprecedented and unique. Sadly, it was also temporary.

God warned the Israelites that His presence would only remain with them in the Temple as long as they followed His law and served Him alone.

> "But if you or your sons indeed turn away from following Me, and do not keep My commandments and My statutes which I have set before you, and go and serve other gods and worship them, then I will cut off Israel from the land which I have given them, and the house which I have consecrated for My name, I will cast out of My sight. So Israel will become a proverb and a byword among all peoples. And this house will become a heap of ruins; everyone who passes by will be astonished and hiss and say, 'Why has the LORD done thus to this land and to this house?' And they will say, 'Because they forsook the LORD their God, who brought their fathers out of the land of Egypt, and adopted other gods and worshiped them and served them, therefore the LORD has brought all this adversity on them.'" 1 Kings 9:6-9 (NASB)

Unfortunately, this warning went unheeded, and God's presence left the Temple a few generations later, reducing the Temple to something like a gleaming, golden movie set, instead of a place to encounter the living God. Eventually even this edifice was destroyed when the Babylonians conquered the apostate Southern Kingdom in 586 B.C. That God would allow such a catastrophe to befall people called by His name and a structure that represented and hosted His glory clearly reveals this: **God is not impressed with the grandness of a physical structure if it comes at the cost of a heart fully given over to Him.**

A New Temple Of Flesh

Thankfully, God did not permanently withdraw His Spirit's presence from our lives because of the unfaithfulness of Israel. He had a better plan.

*"And I will give them one heart, and put a new spirit within them. And I
will take the heart of stone out of their flesh
and give them a heart of flesh" Ezekiel 11:19 (NASB)*

*Gathering them together, He [Jesus] commanded them not to leave Jeru-
salem, but to wait for what the Father had promised, "Which" He said,
"you heard of from Me; for John baptized with water, but you will be
baptized with the Holy Spirit not many days from now."
Acts 1:4-5 (NASB)*

We should care for our physical bodies today because we become repositories
for the Holy Spirit when we experience saving faith in Jesus. God Himself, in the
person of the Holy Spirit, takes up residence in all believers and enables us to live
out the Christ life that would be impossible without His presence.

The Apostle Paul reminds us of this truth in these verses:

*Or do you not know that your body is a temple of the Holy Spirit who is
in you, whom you have from God, and that you are not your own? For
you have been bought with a price: therefore glorify God in your body.
1 Corinthians 6:19-20 (NASB)*

As this verse states, the Holy Spirit's presence isn't like that of a squatter or
even a renter. Jesus bought us with the high price of the cross, and takes possession
of what He purchased by putting His Spirit within us. *The Holy Spirit's presence
in our lives confirms His ownership of our bodies just as He exerted ownership
of the original Temple in Jerusalem.* It is crucial that the pursuer of fitness take
care to build on a temple foundation with materials that will stand a test by fire (1
Corinthians 3).

For the reader who is challenged by this Temple analogy, doesn't it seem a little
incongruous to be possessed by the Spirit of the living God and yet house this
greatness in the equivalent of a dilapidated mobile home? Dilapidated not because
of circumstances beyond our control, but out of sheer neglect? Our current bodies
are temporary and are given to natural decay (2 Corinthians 4:7-18). There is a
difference, however, between the natural aging process and the unnatural destruction so many are bringing on themselves through neglect. Glorifying God with
our bodies is the appropriate response to the incredible reality of God's personal
possession. This should make a dramatic impact on what we *do* with our bodies, as
well as what we *are.*

The opening phrase "or do you not know…" in the Scripture on the previous
page strongly suggests that those in the church at Corinth had forgotten the signifi-

cance of this reality in the midst of a permissive culture. Over 2000 years removed from when this was written, our ignorance is even more profound.

God Doesn't Make Junk

Whether it was the wilderness Tabernacle of Moses' day or Solomon's grand Temple, God's dwelling place was constructed of the finest materials available. Construction and maintenance was not performed as an afterthought replete with bailing wire and duct tape. God Himself put the blueprints together for His earthly dwellings, just as He planned out the ingenious creation of our bodies (God's creative work will be covered in Chapter 13).

The Psalmist understood the miraculous nature of our physical state:

> For You formed my inward parts; You wove me in my mother's womb. I will give thanks to You, for I am fearfully and wonderfully made; wonderful are Your works, and my soul knows it very well. My frame was not hidden from You, When I was made in secret, and skillfully wrought in the depths of the earth; Your eyes have seen my unformed substance; and in Your book were all written The days that were ordained for me.
> Psalms 139: 13- 16 (NASB)

The Apostle Paul further detailed the implications of a Spirit-possessed body for the believers in Rome:

> But if the Spirit of him who raised Jesus from the dead dwells in you, he who raised Christ Jesus from the dead will also give life to your mortal bodies through His Spirit who dwells in you. So then, brethren, we are under obligation, not to the flesh, to live according to the flesh— for if you live according to the flesh, you must die; but if by the Spirit you are putting to death the deeds of the body, you will live. For all who are being led by the Spirit of God, these are the sons of God. For you have not received a spirit of slavery leading to fear again, but you have received a spirit of adoption as sons by which we cry out, 'Abba, Father!' The Spirit Himself testifies with our spirit that we are children of God, and if children, heirs also, heirs of God and fellow heirs with Christ, if indeed we suffer with him so that we may also be glorified with him.
> Romans 8: 11-17 (NASB)

Surrendering Our Bodies To God's Control

James Cameron's film *Avatar* became the highest grossing movie of all time in telling the story of a reluctant military recruit whose mind possesses a creature from another planet. His thoughts, skills, prejudices, and desires have full sway over his otherworldly host. Have you ever considered yourself an avatar for the Holy Spirit? Jesus wants to live His life out through us, exerting authority and control of our minds and bodies. What a battle we wage in so many areas, including the physical, as we bow to God's prerogatives as rightful owner of our lives! Many things can quench or grieve the Holy Spirit and limit His ability to move unfettered through our lives. Unwholesome media, misuse of our tongues, harboring anger, bitterness toward others, etc., are all ways we muzzle the Spirit's activity and attempt to reassert ownership over a life and body that's no longer ours. Despite whatever resistance and obstacles we are erecting, the Spirit is constantly working to produce fruit worthy of the King. Can we honestly say that we are available to produce the fruit of a spirit-possessed life when our physical state works at cross purposes with His ownership and control? After all, self-control makes the short list of primary attributes of a Spirit-directed life.

> *"But the fruit of the Spirit is love, joy, peace, patience, kindness,*
> *goodness, faithfulness, gentleness, **self-control**;*
> *against such things there is no law."Galatians 5:22 -23 (NASB)*

What a privilege we have to know God so intimately! What a challenge to consider the grandeur of the previous hosts of God's glory. How humbling to realize that God is not impressed with the physical image we're projecting to the world, when it is not motivated by and aligned with His Spirit. What a journey we have before us to seek continual transformation of our bodies and spirits so we more closely conform to our creator's intent.

I began this chapter drawing parallels between some circumstances in the life of Susan Boyle and the call we have to balance physical and spiritual priorities. At the audition that set the trajectory of Ms. Boyle's unlikely career she had the audacity, before uttering a note, to suggest to a live and television audience that she would like to follow in the steps of the world-renowned British singer Elaine Page. By the power of the indwelling Holy Spirit, we are to aspire to some nervy heights as well: nothing less than conformity to the image of Jesus.

Our calling in the power of the Holy Spirit is to continuously reduce the gap between our positional standing of physical and spiritual perfection before God and the reality of lives still under construction.

1. *London Daily Mail* August 2, 2010

CHAPTER 10

THE ELEPHANT IN THE ROOM

"I don't know what the deal is!" Mark said with an exasperated edge to his voice. "I'm bustin' my butt in here five days a week and getting nowhere. I keep waiting for a payday that never seems to come!"

It was true. Mark could be found in my gym most weekdays between 5 and 6:30 p.m., his XXL shirt lathered with sweat from lifting weights and a half hour on a treadmill. At thirty years old, he'd clearly worked hard at accumulating nearly 300 pounds on his six-foot frame, but he'd seemingly found a new passion for living and was now putting in the effort necessary to see substantive change. After a quick, encouraging drop of ten pounds, however, Mark's body seemed to cling to its fat like white on rice.

"I was hoping I could avoid going on insulin, but I'm worried what my next checkup is gonna show," he confessed, barely masking his frustration. "My wife isn't happy with the C-Pap mask I wear at night," he added. "And then there's this darn ED...." His voice trailed off and I was sure what I heard was not just disappointment—it was raw pain.

What was I going to say to this guy? I knew how things worked: calories in, calories out. It was clear he was following the workout routines I'd been giving him, and he seemed committed to success. You could see the enthusiasm on his face in the early days of his club membership; like a man invigorated by a new and worthwhile cause. His body language said something different now ... shoulders slumped, an elbow hanging limply on the corner of my desk, and his eyes boring a hole in the well-worn linoleum floor.

"Are you following the meal plan I gave you?" I asked, knowing that his food intake was the unknown factor in this puzzling equation. "Pretty much," he replied. "I can't do it perfect all the time, of course, but I've worked on cuttin' down."

I pressed him. "What, exactly, have you done to follow the meal plan we went over last month?"

Unaccustomed to modest accountability, Mark seemed taken aback. He momentarily blanched before stammering, "Like I said … I've been cuttin' back."

I abruptly stood up, taking him by surprise. "Let's go out to your car", I offered on a hunch. Mark began to form a verbal protest but I was already opening the office door and making my way into the gym lobby. Energetic music was pulsating through the club, but I could still hear him trying to construct a response as he shouldered his gym bag and reluctantly followed me out the door.

"You're in the red Malibu, right?" I shot over my shoulder as I stepped off the curb into the lot.

"Um ... yeah …" he stuttered, still trying to process what was happening.

Mark's car was hard to miss with its mud-caked undercarriage and filthy windows. The car screamed "wash me." In many respects it was a metaphor for his life: unkempt on the outside and likely harboring debilitating secrets within.

As we neared his vehicle, the back peddling began in earnest. "Y'know, I still enjoy a burger for lunch now and again … and they've just started up again with those dang shakes in my favorite flavor. What are we doing out here anyway?"

I turned again to face Mark as I reached the rear driver's side door of his four-door sedan. "The kind of car a person drives says a lot about their personality. The exterior often tells me how they feel about themselves. On the other hand, the inside of a person's car often tells me if they're following my meal plan."

My raised palm was extended toward him in a silent request for his keys.

"Aw … hell …" he muttered under his breath and I heard two beeps from his remote key as he turned away and looked absently into the sky. I swung open the passenger door and for a moment understood the thrill of a paleontologist arriving at an archeological dig. I was greeted by layers of fast-food sacks, french fry cartons, pop cans, energy drinks, candy wrappers, and potato chip bags. Each stratum gave silent testimony to his dietary activity the past several weeks.

"What are you doing, Mark?" I asked, letting the question hang in the air unanswered for several moments. I finally broke the uncomfortable silence. "You came to me a couple of months ago fed up with what you had become. I explained to you this would take hard work and wouldn't resolve itself in a week or two, but would be a long-term strategy."

"I remember," was all he could muster.

"Think of this as an investment. When you come into the gym and put in a good workout, you're putting money in your account. Same for following the meal plan we've put together—that's another deposit toward your investment goal. What I'm seeing here in your car represents massive withdrawals of all the deposits you're making, leaving you with no account balance. You're just treading water."

"Change is hard, Joe. I'm not like you."

"We've all got our baggage, Mark," I said, trying to strike a conciliatory tone. "Somehow you're going to have to catch a vision of what you can become, and in doing so decide that hard sacrifices now are worth a great payoff in the future."

— — — — — — — — — — — — — — —

I wish I could say that our conversation that day was a game-changer for Mark, but the truth is that despite a level of desire for change, his destructive dietary tendencies continued to sabotage his progress. Over several years, my work with him got him off insulin three times. He's lost the same 100 pounds three times as well. After a long absence, I ran into Mark at a restaurant and was saddened to see him tucking away a large pile of chicken wings and washing it down with several beers.

I didn't bother looking in his car as I left.

What's Your Motivation?

As a personal trainer and nutrition counselor, stories like Mark's are common. In Part Four of this book—**Foundation**—David will develop the principal of sowing and reaping. To be sure, Mark had been sowing seeds of his own destruction even as I tried to warn him of the onerous compound interest he would inevitably pay. As I encourage people toward life change, I appeal to their desire to feel better. I remind them of the financial costs they're facing now and will certainly fork over in the future. When the relationship allows, I'll even appeal to their motherhood or fatherhood, asking if they want to be around to see their sons or daughters graduate from college. Tough love, I know, but the truth is that the obituary page in our local paper is filled with men and women in their fifties and sixties who have no business dying that young. Our hospitals and pharmacies are filled with many more who are resigning themselves to a quality of life far below what should be theirs.

Over the years, literally thousands of clients have told me about their desire to improve their physical health. Some have been sowing bad seeds for decades and are desperate for a second chance just as the compound interest for their life investments comes due. Others recognize at an earlier stage that fundamental changes are necessary. The good news is there's always an opportunity to turn things around, if a decision is made to begin sowing good seed.

The elephant in the room during my one-on-one client meetings is this: *Why are you really here?*

Are you seeking help at a fitness center or through this book because a recent medical checkup has you momentarily scared? Are you appeasing your husband or wife? Are you hoping physical changes will fill the spiritual void in your life? Are you looking for compliments that will feed your ego? Or are you here because you have a deep conviction that your present lifestyle is unacceptable and unsustainable, and you're ready to do what's necessary to start sowing seeds toward a preferable return?

How you answer these questions will almost certainly mean the difference between long-term success and temporary improvements that eventually disappear as you revert back to familiar life habits. So I have to ask: *Why are you really here?* The contents of this book will provide a road map for positive change. Your answer to that question will decide whether it lasts.

Because your mind, body, and spirit are intertwined, sorting out motivations is complicated. But as a follower of Jesus, you have a distinct advantage as you face hard questions about yourself. Understanding that there is a spiritual component to address, and letting the light of truth inform your decisions gives you every chance of reaching your goal. You can be distracted, foolish, ignorant, and unconcerned about your physical state for a long time and still redeem your later years, if you will do some soul searching and come to a place of deep conviction.

Tracy's story is an example of this kind of redemption.

A believing, middle-aged pharmacy tech at my church, Tracy had every reason to avoid the struggles of those she had seen with serious illness. She had watched her mother, who had adult-onset diabetes, struggle with the inconvenience and limitations of an insulin-dependent life. At work, Tracy saw the increasing number of people diagnosed with diabetes as they purchased insulin and test strips from her pharmacy. Tracy understood the costs of this condition. But as the years went by and the pounds went on, she ignored reality by avoiding a simple blood test.

Unable to put it off forever, Tracy went to her doctor for a physical and was routinely informed by phone that a prescription for diabetic supplies would be called into her pharmacy. "That's it?" she wondered to herself, "That's how this goes down? No alternatives? Just pick up your supplies?" Sobered by the cost of the hole she'd dug for herself, she began to identify her core issue as a spiritual one— idolatry. Wasn't she constantly thinking about food? Wasn't she always thinking about a recipe or what she was going to make for dinner tomorrow and the night after and the night after? An honest look at her thought life put food squarely in the starring role. She had made it her idol—her god.

Knowing this was unacceptable for a believer, Tracy began making changes to her diet, her schedule, her study, prayer life, and her physical activity. As a result, her thought life began reforming. Life no longer revolved around the next meal, the new recipe, and the pleasure of food.

Tracy has been sowing a different kind of seed for months now, and she's reaping a wonderful physical and spiritual harvest. It's a particularly wonderful harvest because it doesn't include diabetic supplies.

PART FOUR

FOUNDATIONS

CHAPTER 11

LIFE LESSONS FROM FLYOVER COUNTRY

The early months of my relationship with my wife, Beth, were filled with long separations and frequent travel. After meeting on a mission trip to Japan, we headed back to our home states, wondering if this budding romance was over before it started or if it could be sustained through correspondence and air travel (If you can imagine it, we survived in a world with no email, Facebook, or Skype). Beth visited me in Southern California first, and I reciprocated with an extended Labor Day weekend trip to her native central Iowa—the first of many during our long-distance courtship, which lasted nearly two years.

Coming from Orange County, where the orange trees and strawberry farms had been nearly eradicated by concrete, I was visually struck by my bird's-eye view as I landed in Des Moines: *Everything was so green.* While my early years were spent in central California's fertile San Joaquin Valley, the olive and citrus groves I grew up with didn't have the visual impact that thousands of acres of corn, soybeans, and hay did that day. With its tractors, seed commercials on TV, and other signs of farm work, it was obvious from the start that agriculture was a dominant presence in a state where the slogan at the time was "A Place to Grow."

Since moving to Des Moines in 1988 after marriage, I've learned that its agricultural roots have blended with growing insurance and financial services industry, adding an incongruous urban white collar to the bib overalls common just past the city limits. It's from these two disciplines—agriculture and finance—that we learn trustworthy biblical principles that speak directly to our physical lives.

Agriculture meets finance

Sowing and reaping and *compound return* are foundational truths that are not only familiar to every Iowa farmer and insurance-company actuary, they're also woven into biblical texts as well as each of our life stories. These laws are objective realities that impact all of us in the financial, social, and physical arenas of our lives. The Book of Job, probably the earliest-written book in the Bible and one of antiquities' oldest writings, speaks to the immutable truths of *sowing and reaping.*

> *"As I have seen, those who plow iniquity and sow trouble reap the same." Job 4:8 (ESV)*

The wisest man who ever lived spoke on this principle as well.

> *"Whoever sows injustice will reap calamity, and the rod of his fury will fail." Proverbs 22:8 (ESV)*

The Apostle Paul reminds the church in Galatia that they ignore this principle at their own peril.

> *"Do not be deceived: God is not mocked, for whatever one sows, that will he also reap. For the one who sows to his own flesh will from the flesh reap corruption, but the one who sows to the Spirit will from the Spirit reap eternal life." Galatians 6:7-8 (ESV)*

If you live past your teens, you begin to understand the truth of sowing and reaping in your own experience.

- If you don't study or do the your homework, you receive poor test scores.
- If you don't invest in relationships, life will get lonely in times of crisis.
- If you don't work out over the summer, the first week of football or cross-country running will not be a pleasant experience.
- If you save your allowance and lawn-mowing earnings, you'll have money when you find an item you really want to buy.

In young adulthood, yet more facets of this truth are discovered.

- High school academics have implications for your success in college.

- Relationships nurtured in high school and college often become invaluable when looking for an internship, a summer job, or a permanent vocation.

- High school jocks and college socialites who major in sports and parties often find that their degrees don't translate into fulfilling careers.

- Saving money now helps you avoid paying later on high-interest-rate credit cards.

Closely related to sowing and reaping is the principle of compound return. This precept teaches that small, incremental steps or contributions end up yielding an oversized return over time. The Old and New Testaments speak about compound return as both a law of nature as well as spiritual truth.

For they sow the wind, and they shall reap the whirlwind. Hosea 8:7 (ESV)

Because I have called and you refused to listen, have stretched out my hand and no one has heeded, because you have ignored all my counsel and would have none of my reproof, I also will laugh at your calamity; I will mock when terror strikes you, when terror strikes you like a storm and calamity comes like a whirlwind, when distress and anguish come upon you Proverbs 1:24-27 (ESV)

A little sleep, a little slumber, a little folding of the hands to rest, and poverty will come upon you like a robber, and want like an armed man. Proverbs 6: 10-11 (ESV)

"Everyone who comes to Me and hears My words and does them, I will show you what he is like: he is like a man building a house, who dug deep and laid the foundation on the rock. And when a flood arose, the stream broke against that house and could not shake it, because it had been well built. But the one who hears and does not do them is like a man who built a house on the ground without any foundation. When the stream broke against it, immediately it fell, and the ruin of that house was great."— Jesus speaking in Luke 6:47-49 (ESV)

"Bring the whole tithe into the storehouse, so that there may be food in My house, and test Me now in this," says the Lord of hosts, "if I will not open for you the windows of heaven, and pour out for you a blessing until it overflows." Malachi 3:10 (NASB)

Before the financial crises that began in 2008, a saver was able to earn a decent return placing money in an interest-bearing savings account or money-market account. Over a period of many years, even a small investment in financial instruments like these could multiply into something substantial. During the last few years of these long-term investments, the power of compounding interest is especially evident, going almost parabolic as it surges in value. Like a seed of corn that has been dormant under the soil for weeks only to explode to over seven feet tall in a matter of three months, large returns can come from small, regular investments. The Scriptures above, as well as life experience, reveals that faithful and wise life investments provide an abundant return. Poor or insufficient investments—or no investments at all—lead to sudden, often tragic consequences.

These principles are at work through several high-profile examples in the Old Testament. The High Priest Eli, while sharing words of wisdom with the young Samuel, allowed his own sons to grievously abuse their positions of authority over many years, leading to a calamitous and sudden end in 1 Samuel chapter 4. King David's sin with Bathsheba and his festering relationship with son Absalom came to a sudden crisis in 2 Samuel 15-17. On a positive note, Joseph's many years of unrecognized faithfulness and stewardship was rewarded in the span of a single day in Genesis 41. In Mark 10:29-31 is one of many examples where Jesus speaks to the exceedingly generous interest His Father pays to those who invest liberally in the Kingdom of God.

The principles of sowing and reaping, and compound return are played out not only on the pages of Scripture; I've seen them at work throughout my life, as well.

During my career as an ice cream salesman and executive, my sales manager Randy and I regularly trekked thirty-five minutes north of Des Moines to Ames, the home of Iowa State University. In addition to the university, which was a large ice cream buyer, Ames also boasted the state's largest restaurant purchaser of ice cream. I can't tell you how many times we hobnobbed with the ISU Purchasing Department personnel and lunched at the enormous barbecue restaurant. We developed relationships, determined needs, and secured their trust. Back at the office, we custom-formulated products and packaging, and took a sharp pencil to our prices. We sowed seeds. Seeds that lay dormant for months before becoming fruitful.

When at last our months of seed-sowing reaped a harvest of business, the compounded return to our bulk ice cream business was staggering. Nearly overnight, our little ice cream company became a major regional player in institutional ice cream sales, having secured the state's two largest bulk ice cream customers. The satisfaction we enjoyed from our hard-earned success was worth the substantial time and effort we invested, and the boost this new business brought allowed us to better serve our existing customers and be more competitive securing new ones.

Years later, within a few months of my leaving the company, I was saddened to hear that we'd lost the Ames restaurant business to a competitor. Seeing an opportunity, they had been sowing seed of their own. The loss of business came as a bitter and sobering reminder that sowing, reaping, and compound return have both positive and negative outcomes.

You can point to many examples in your own life where the principles of sowing and reaping, as well as compound return, have left their inevitable mark. Hopefully most are positive and you are enjoying the fruit of your investments. *Here is a strange thing, however: These principles, which are readily accepted in financial, relational, and educational spheres, are often ignored in the physical and health realm, where our daily choices will impact a future harvest. Consider these inevitable consequences:*

- The high school student who has not learned self-restraint while eating at home in preparation for the new, buffet-style dining format at college,

- The active college student who discounts the exercise-free routines that emerge post-marriage as insignificant lifestyle adjustments,

- The pregnant mom who gives in to every craving with the justification that she'll shed all her "baby-weight" once she delivers,

- The busy father of young children who becomes content to watch on the sidelines and reminisce about his days in organized sports,

- The middle-aged traveling regional manager who eats drive-thru meals each weekday between accounts and feels his expanding waistline is a lost cause,

- The administrative assistant who develops a weekday ritual of pastry washed down with a latte—and calls it breakfast,

- The couple who snack away the evenings together while wondering why their clothes keep shrinking.

We intuitively know that our actions set the stage for ramifications down the road. That's why so many save their money, invest in relationships, and obey the law. Why then is it that, despite all the information we have at our disposal, we serially ignore its wisdom? Why do so many live as if they'll be the exception that will cheat death and avoid the inevitable consequences of their lifestyle?

One of my former pastors was fond of saying about the challenges of marriage,

"Marriage is a challenge because it's so *daily*." Indeed, the *daily* nature of our food and activity choices presents daily opportunities to either surrender our desire for immediate gratification to a higher call of Kingdom availability and worship or to sow seeds for a different kind of harvest.

Allure of the Quick Fix

In our culture, many of us refuse to take personal responsibility for our health, and succumb to the siren song of the quick fix. We have become so trustful of our health-care system that we believe it will be capable of rescuing us from whatever physical trial we will inevitably face.

Do you have a consistent lack of energy and feel lethargic? Grab an energy drink to get you through the morning/afternoon/evening. High blood pressure? High cholesterol? Joint pain? High blood sugar? Depression? Why deal with the causes when you can just get a prescription. A family history of heart attacks and strokes? Don't change your lifestyle— just put your order in for a stent, balloon procedure, or bypass surgery.

While our advances in medicine have allowed us to often mitigate the principle of compound return when we have sowed poorly and are set to reap a bitter harvest, this approach has a spiritual dimension that must be addressed by all followers of Jesus.

After squandering our life's income on consumption, do we rightly expect someone else to give us a comfortable retirement? After a lifetime of alienating our family by our behavior, do we expect them to rally to our side in our time of need? After repeatedly violating laws, do we expect authorities to cut us a break because we don't want to face the consequences?

The answers to these rhetorical questions may seem self-evident. *Of course we have to except the consequences of our behavior.* **In the arena of health, however, we're often given the option of passing the costs of our lifestyle choices on to someone else.** While "sowing the wind" and letting someone else "reap the whirlwind" is a natural fleshly inclination, it's hard to square with admonitions to love our neighbor as ourselves. Even with modern medicine, there are many occasions when medical miracles can't save us and we do personally reap what we've sown. Then there's only the question of what we've stolen from our families, churches, and communities through our absence.

- - - - - - - - - - - - - - - -

Little did I know that the green farmland and bustling city I surveyed from 10,000 feet all those years ago would become the place I'd call home for the past twenty-six years. The lessons of the land and the financial services industry have remained relevant and true all that time. Sowing, reaping, and compound interest in the area of personal fitness has afforded my family many great experiences: fifteen-mile family hikes at altitude in Colorado; long (and often treacherous) mountain bike rides with my boys through forest trails; white-water rafting as a family down the Arkansas river in Colorado, and weight lifting at the health club for school sports conditioning. All these are fond memories for my entire family. During the early years of our marriage, the full-yield potential of these seeds lay dormant. But Beth and I continued sowing through myriad daily decisions because we believed in the principles I've described in this chapter. We're still sowing. But increasingly we're beginning to reap as well.

A few months ago, my twenty-one-year-old son asked me if I wanted to go running with him. He'd been training for a 10 K run at college and wanted to stay on schedule while home for a break. Since running was a regular part of my own fitness regimen, I complied, glad for the chance to do something active together. After the brisk five-mile course was completed, he turned to me and said, "You know, it's pretty cool that I can go on a long, hard run with my dad. I don't know any of my friends who would be able to experience that."

In that moment, I'd have to say that compound interest felt really good.

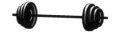

CHAPTER 12

FOUNDATIONAL FITNESS

Becoming healthy and fit is not a mysterious experience that can only be under-stood and enjoyed by a few with access to inside information. For the most part, the many benefits of a fit life are the fruit of common sense, self-control, a willingness to move, and an awareness of the numerous traps our culture presents to derail us.

Like most other products and services, healthy living has become a marketable commodity. This has engendered confusion, largely due to all the competing voices and options that claim to have the best means to this end. Promoting and marketing a healthy lifestyle has only entered our vocabulary in recent decades. Though health and wellness has long had its proponents, consumers in the 1960s and earlier were not continually bombarded with advertisements and products promising an easy path to fitness.

My role in this book is to give you basic, sound, and practical information as you begin to implement a strategy for better health. This chapter will lay the foundation for that pursuit, and future chapters will add greater detail to this basic framework.

The Five Building Blocks

There are five building blocks that comprise foundational fitness and, because they are derived from common sense, I'm going to use the acronym **SENSE** to help you remember these blocks:

S: Strength. Building lean muscle

E: Eating. Building awareness of your calorie intake

N: Nutrition. Assuring proper nutrition

S: Support. Coaching and accountability

E: Exercise. Cardiovascular conditioning

All of these important elements work in concert with each other. I hope you will see the synergy that is developed when they are all utilized as a package. Whether you are badly deconditioned or training for competitive purposes, these five areas remain at the core of everything you will do in the physical realm.

Strength

Weight-bearing exercise, or resistance training, is one of the least understood aspects of foundational fitness. Often viewed as an extra only pursued by serious fitness devotees, this discipline is far more integral to success than you might imagine. The average person didn't look to strength conditioning a couple of generations ago due to ignorance of its benefits. Also, heavy lifting was integrated into the lives of most people as they went about their daily routines. Before plastics, fiberglass, silicon, veneers, foam board, and other lightweight materials, nearly everything that people moved, carried, pushed, or pulled weighed more than similar objects today and took more effort to transport. Before escalators, elevators, 15-speed bikes, moving walkways, mopeds, and hydraulics, traveling and dealing with the basics of life involved lots of resistance training. In today's world, developing sufficient muscle tissue requires a plan. We lose one percent of our muscle mass per year as we age, so developing a "muscle reservoir" and maintaining it has become important as we approach middle age and beyond.

The athlete looking to improve his or her performance and the individual seeking to shed excess weight must make an effort in this area. Whenever the topic of weight-lifting is broached, mental images are usually evoked of burly men hoisting iron plates. For the serious athlete this will be a reality, but for most people the hindrance this intimidating vision provides needs to be replaced.

The purpose of resistance training is to build lean muscle tissue, and there are many ways to do this including bands, isometric exercises (bearing only your own weight), inflatable balls, smaller dumbbells, free weights, and machines. The benefits of greater lean muscle tissue include improved strength and flexibility, a decreased risk of osteoporosis (weakening of bones), and rapid burning of calories. *Muscle tissue is where the body burns calories, and it burns up to ten times more calories than fat tissue! Muscle tissue that is built and sustained through proper nutrition will make you a fat-burning machine when you are active and you will continue to burn more calories even at rest.*

Because they are familiar, running on treadmills, climbing stairs, and similar activities are favored by many when starting fitness routines. But you need strength training too. Seek help from a competent trainer or knowledgeable friend if you try unfamiliar weight-bearing exercises that develop certain muscle groups. Don't let your unfamiliarity keep you from making strength training a consistent part of your weekly fitness routine!

Detailed pictorial information regarding muscle groups, specific lifting exercises, etc. are available through our website, *www.fit4theking.net.*

Eating

Food intake is foundational to fitness, obviously. Future chapters on nutrition will go into more detail. For now, I'd like to concentrate on what you eat, how much we eat, and how this impacts your weight.

First, a science lesson. The First Law of Thermodynamics states that energy is neither created nor destroyed; it only changes form. "Calorie" is a term that quantifies the amount of energy in food. One calorie is the amount of energy required to raise the temperature of one gram of water by one degree Celsius. In layman's terms, calories are simply a measurement of energy that is being expended to fuel your body.

Aside from water or water-based beverages, everything you consume has a caloric value. Calories are not evil. They don't have a moral component. What does have a moral component is choosing to consistently consume an unhealthy excess of calories without nutritional consideration. These are often described as "empty calories," which means calories without nutritional benefit to your body. These kinds of calories are generally inexpensive, readily available, and at the core of our national eating disorder.

Every body is unique, and we all need a differing amount of calories each day to fuel our bodies. The rate at which your body burns energy is called your metabolic rate, and when you're at rest it's called your Basal Metabolic Rate (BMR). Our body structure (muscle mass, bone density, etc.), our activity levels, our sex, and even our sleeping patterns affect our metabolism. Any intake of calories beyond what you burn through movement and body function is called your caloric surplus. Over time, the surplus adds layers of unhealthy and mobility-limiting fat to your body. This fat is stored fuel, basically, sitting in reserve for when it is converted to usable energy. Conversely, any activity that burns more calories than you're consuming is called your caloric deficit. When your body needs extra calories, it gets them from your stored fat. For those desiring to lose fat, it will be necessary to achieve a caloric deficit by both increasing activity and/or reducing consumption. Achieving this goal without robbing your body of the nutrition needed to function well will be covered in the *Nutrition* chapters that follow.

These facts about how our bodies uniquely metabolize food reveal why we need to take personal responsibility for our intake as well as why one-size-fits-all diets don't work. Our culture presents nutritional information and portion sizes without consideration of the individual's needs. What do I mean by this? The "Personal

Pan Pizza" may be a reasonable meal for one person and a meal and a half for another. The 16-ounce beverage served with a meal might be appropriate for one person and not another. The "suggested serving size" or meal portion at a restaurant cannot be appropriate for everyone. More likely than not, the portion you're being offered is larger than your body needs to sustain itself, to say nothing of its nutritional content.

Two basic questions need to be considered any time we're consuming food and drink. *First, how many calories do I need to sustain my body so that it performs optimally?* An understanding of your metabolic rate is crucial here (to calculate your BMR, visit our website). *Second, how much nutritional value is present in the calories I'm consuming?* Am I eating with a purpose or just consuming food without nutritional consideration?

These questions may sound legalistic and constrictive to many. Who wants to count calories and read nutrition labels? But they are necessary if you want to discover the unique equilibrium of consumption and activity that leads you to a healthy weight. Once you establish eating habits that predominantly include nutrient-dense foods, you won't need to worry about labels and calorie counts because you will be eating within a zone of safety. Previous generations did not have to plan or strategize their eating to the degree we must today because sound food choices were readily available. For proof, look at the obesity epidemic we are experiencing in this country. Ironically, despite the overload of calories we're consuming, many remain nutritionally deficient.

In an effort to help with basic portion control, here is a guideline that many have found helpful: it's called MyPlate (*www.choosemyplate.gov*). It's the government's replacement for the outdated and carbohydrate-heavy Food Pyramid. The focus of MyPlate is portion control. For instance, a MyPlate meal includes a portion of protein that is roughly the size of the palm of your hand. While this protein will usually be some kind of meat, it could also be a serving of quinoa, a combination of rice and beans, cottage cheese, or other good protein sources. Along with the meat portion, select a quality carbohydrate that is roughly the same size as your protein portion. Examples of quality carbohydrates are yams/sweet potatoes, 100 percent whole grain bread, brown rice, and whole wheat pasta.

The remaining two portions should be fruits and vegetables, and they should comprise the majority of your plate. Fresh fruits and vegetables are best, and the darker green and more colorful they are, the more likely they possess higher levels of important nutrients. Dairy products are another essential food group and can be included via a milk beverage, yogurt, or cottage cheese. Your average microwavable meal or restaurant selection will almost certainly not resemble a balanced MyPlate meal. Yet restaurant meals have become the norm for many who are overweight and undernourished.

The MyPlate approach is designed to work with the normal rhythms of our culture, which is accustomed to three meals per day. Ideally, you would take these three meals and break them up into five smaller meals consumed about every three hours. By giving your body consistent intakes of nutrition, your metabolic rate will be elevated. This keeps your brain from signaling starvation, which often leads to overconsumption.

Both David and I have gravitated toward core foods that we think taste great, are reasonably convenient, affordable, and loaded with nutrition. Because we consistently choose appropriate portions from this list, we don't count calories. We are eating healthy foods that are supporting fit bodies. To give you practical examples of what fills our plates, here is a list of most of the foods we consume weekly, year in and year out:

Protein (repairs, rebuilds, and grows muscles):
Chicken and turkey breasts
Salmon, tilapia, and tuna
Lean cuts of beef
Pork tenderloins or "America's Cut" of pork
Quinoa
Skim and low-fat white or chocolate milk, low-fat cottage cheese, Greek yogurt
Eggs (mostly whites)
Various nuts (almonds, cashews, pecans, pistachios, and walnuts)

Carbohydrates (energy source):
Bran
Oatmeal (prefer old-fashioned steel cut)
Homemade granola
100 percent whole grain bread
Potatoes (white or red)
Sweet potatoes/yams
Brown rice
Whole wheat pasta
Popcorn

Fruits (fiber, energy source, and loaded with phytonutrients):
Mangoes
Kiwi
Blueberries
Strawberries
Raspberries
Blackberries
Apples
Grapes
Pineapple
Dates

Vegetables (fiber, vitamins, minerals, and loaded with phytonutrients):
Broccoli
Asparagus
Spinach
Red leaf and romaine lettuce
Squash
Corn
Green beans
Edamame
Carrots
Tomatoes
Peas
Beets

Fats and Oils (brain function and heart health):
Olive oil (room temperature)
Avocado
Nut butters
Butter

From among the thousands of food items that are available to us, David and I eat from the above list for probably 85 percent of our caloric intake. This forms the core of our intake because these are nutritionally dense, calorically balanced, and simply delicious foods. The other 15 percent of our caloric intake includes salad dressings, sauces, bread, baked goods, cheese, condiments, sweeteners, tortillas, ice cream, frozen yogurt, chocolate, and more. These extras fill the aisles of the typical grocery store. Our activity level—assuming our weight is under control and our nutritional needs have been met—gives us the freedom to eat small portions of these kinds of nutrient-lite or higher-fat items. There are few hard lines we draw regarding what we won't eat, but it is rare to find us drinking sugared soda, diet soda or sports drinks and eating fast food, donuts, hot dogs, brats, cakes, cookies, and chips. Honestly, if our society experienced a significant reduction in consumption of these products, our national health would improve overnight.

Nutrition

In your effort to lose weight, many reading this book will face the necessity of significantly reducing your consumption. It's imperative that, as you reduce your caloric intake, you meet the nutritional needs of your body. We highly recommended you increase—vigorously, if your health allows—your physical activity as part of your health plan, which makes it even more critical that you eat properly to repair and rebuild your body. If you have not been involved in a regular exercise program, the stresses these changes will place on your body may be significant, and just cutting back on your overall calories without a supplementation plan will limit your results.

Your goal is to starve the fat, feed your muscle, and keep your energy level high enough to support all your other activities. During periods when you are limiting food consumption and shedding weight, low-calorie or calorie-free nutrients are critical. Vitamins, minerals, amino acids, and lean protein sources need to be abundantly available as you transform your body.

There is no shortage of products purporting to help in this effort. We have our favorites, but taking a good multivitamin and a source of supplemental protein/ meal replacement are advised, at a minimum.

Support

Becoming fit, especially if it involves significant weight loss, is not a go-it-alone affair. Most commercial programs that experience any lasting success operate within a group setting or involve personal coaching and accountability. It is no accident that the significant weight loss experienced by people on TV shows like "The Biggest Loser" occurs only with intensive coaching, encouragement, and accountability. As is the case with pursuing any worthy goal, the obstacles to achieving needed weight loss are many, and the journey will be made more enjoyable and sustainable when others are involved.

The power of publicly proclaiming your desire to become healthy, as well as acknowledging past mistakes, has been proven effective by numerous addiction and recovery programs. The veil of shame and secrecy that surrounds any kind of dietary imbalance is lifted when we confess our weakness to others and enlist them in support of change. The phrase "When sin is exposed, it loses its power" has been true in overcoming issues in my life, and it is applicable here. For some, overcoming eating disorders and restoring dietary balance will be similar to overcoming addictions to other substances. Spiritual support and encouragement, accountability, tough love, and celebrating victories are only possible within a community of like-minded people. While attending public forums provides opportunities to share your faith journey as you pursue greater fitness, forming or finding a support group at your church assures that biblical principles and motivations will prevail.

While being a part of a special accountability group can be invaluable in achieving success, it shouldn't come at the expense of the support group most of us have available to us: our families. If you are struggling to find balance and develop healthy eating and exercise habits, it's quite likely others in your family are as well.

Make your activity and meals part of the family conversation. Plan your weekly menus and snacks together. Go to the grocery store together. Educate yourselves together so that one individual isn't carrying the entire emotional, physical, and motivational load. There are few family experiences that have more capacity to promote bonding than this opportunity to "do life" together. While David and I are not prepared to declare complete success as yet, our family conversations about food and fitness, underscored by being good examples at home, have produced a heightened awareness regarding fitness among our children thus far.

Exercise

In an age of modern transportation and technology, opportunities to move and elevate your heart rate often need to be scheduled and sought out. Unless you have a job that provides sustained periods of rhythmic activity, you will need to strategize how you can begin to incorporate activity into your lifestyle. For many, exercise comes with the negative baggage of breathlessness, burning lungs and throat, and even nausea. While shortness of breath and fatigue will always be part of vigorous exercise, negative associations need to be balanced with the overall improvement you feel after you invest in cardiorespiratory training.

What you do to elevate your heart rate is not as important as making the determination to do something. In addition to the obvious options of walking, running, and biking are choices such as rollerblading, trampoline, elliptical machines, jumping rope, group classes, swimming, and stair climbing. The critical issue is choosing exercises that are intense enough to raise your heart rate for a sustained period of time.

Starting slow and building toward more speed, distance, and time is the best strategy. This will prevent early discouragement from aches, pains, and even injury, if you are too aggressive at the start of a regimen.

Walking briskly for less than thirty minutes is probably not going to cut it. Jogging, swimming, and sessions on elliptical machines should last twenty minutes or more. *It is the sustained nature of your elevated heart rate that is going to burn calories, develop endurance, and move your body to a new level of functioning.*

You will notice that I have not advocated some unique and extreme workout regimen here as I've addressed Foundational Fitness. Neither have I suggested that you consume some exotic berry, buy a juicer or food dehydrator, go vegan, or set a goal of climbing Mount Kilimanjaro in the next twelve months. These things will be a part of some people's pursuit of a healthy lifestyle. For most of you, however, consistently experiencing more mainstream and modest changes will enable you to see the benefits from new routines and practices. Though competitive sports are growing in popularity, few of you will be training for a triathlon. Don't let the fact that you're not training for a gold medal keep you from embracing the common sense practices I've covered here that will move you toward becoming *Fit For The King*!

CHAPTER 13
As It Was In The Beginning ...

My eldest son, Austin, has just begun attending medical school, and it's been interesting over the past couple of years to see how his responses have changed during dinner table conversation. Formerly simple questions or statements now receive a more thorough analysis. An innocuous comment by my wife, Beth, about cramping up during her morning run was previously met with only my sympathetic but somewhat trite, "Sorry to hear that, honey." With Austin at the table, we're now treated to a more complex response:

"Your muscles are cramping due to depletion of ions caused by an increase in perspiration during exercise. If you consumed more fluids before you run, especially something with electrolytes, you would be less likely to deplete the ions, which aid in muscle contraction and therefore limit cramping."

A complaint about allergic reactions at his younger brother's landscaping job precipitates this:

"Your mast cells are secreting histamines as they try to deal with the influx of allergens. Your immune system b-cells manufacture a number of IgE [immunoglobulins] that will, in turn, cause the mast cells to release histamines during the cascading process of an allergic reaction. Using Benadryl will help to break down the histamines leading to inflammation and other symptoms."

I'm reminded in these exchanges that we inhabit amazing, complex, integrated, intelligently-designed bodies. While there have clearly been adaptations and mutations along the way that helped humans survive and thrive, the evolutionary theory has always impressed me as a belief that provides supposed scientific cover for a personal philosophy that does not want to acknowledge a Creator. Call me simplistic, but the more we discover about our bodies, the more clear it becomes to me that *I was put together on purpose and for a purpose.*

The Purpose For Our Creation

The Bible doesn't deal in test tubes and petri dishes in describing our creation. Genesis 1 tells us that man was created from dust, and woman was formed from

God's prototype. While God spoke everything else into existence, He used existing materials to create Adam and Eve. This is not the only uniqueness we possess. While all His previous works—the celestial universe, plants, animals, fish, earth, and water—were pronounced "good," mankind was pronounced "very good." There was clearly something about God's creative finale that was unprecedented and exceptional.

Unlike all the earlier created objects and beings, we alone possessed the *imago Dei*—the image of God. Much has been written about exactly what this entails, including whether or not this included physical, spiritual, or intellectual attributes— or all three. Several things are clear, however. When humankind arrived on the scene, *we were more like the Godhead than any previous part of God's creation.*

Artists through the centuries have created renderings of what they imagine Adam and Eve looked like physically. Their paintings tend to reflect notions of beauty and body composition that were attractive at the time. Thus, these artists, most European, created Adam and Eve *in their own image*, including fair skin and dimpled cheeks.

Museum paintings aside, I think it's important to consider what Adam and Eve might have actually looked like based on facts we know, not cultural interpretations. I'm not necessarily talking about skin color, length of hair, or the size of their noses, but I want to focus on their body compositions. Like any designer who is creating a model, God had a purposeful vision in mind when He created man and woman. Clearly, they would be a reflection of their Creator, just as His previous creations were. [1] Beyond that, they were given tasks to perform that would have influenced their physical features. I believe what God created in Adam and Eve could be considered His *ideal prototype*, with physical characteristics He desired to see replicated in the generations to follow.

What were God's stated purposes for Adam and Eve? Genesis 1 and 2 describes the following tasks God commanded the man and woman to perform:

— Cultivate and maintain their Garden

— Subdue and rule over the earth

— Name the animals (Adam)

— Procreate

— Feed themselves

— Care for Eve (Adam)

— Help Adam (Eve)

— Obey and enjoy God

100

After destroying most life in the Flood, God essentially reiterates the same list of commands to Noah and his family after disembarking from the Ark (Genesis 8 and 9). While there certainly wasn't much detail to this list, these are the stripped-down basics. It's interesting to notice that all but the naming of animals calls for a clear physical response. Anyone who's tended a garden or performed landscaping work knows that even with power equipment, this is physical work. While they might not have considered procreating to be *work* per se, this, too, is an *activity* necessitating a healthy, functioning body. God would have given bodies to Adam and Eve that were capable of fulfilling the tasks He assigned them. Suffice to say, these were *big* assignments.

There is something to be gleaned as well from the structure of the week God instituted. In His creative work, He set aside a Sabbath day of rest, during which labor ceased. His clear intention and our assumption should be that God created us with the capacity and responsibility to be actively at work the other six days. Adam and Eve were created with the ability and expectation they would be involved in physical work six days out of every seven.

Implications Of Our Creation

While it would be easy to pass over this history as familiar territory, I believe there are some important takeaways for us as it informs our thinking about God's intentions regarding our physical bodies. Like the rest of creation, God created his ideal prototypes in Adam and Eve. And from what we know so far, these prototypes were the only creations on earth designed in God's image and given the physically demanding task of exercising dominion here. I think it's also safe to assume they did not need a few drinks, flickering candles, an aphrodisiac, or some kind of pill to be physically and sexually attracted to each other.

When you picture the human precedents God conceived ... His ideal ... what comes to mind? Do they resemble most of humanity you see on a daily basis?

What many of us need is a reasonable framework or point of reference regarding God's intentions for our physical bodies as the One who ultimately gives us life. We might not have been created from dust or a rib, but we are each unique, purposeful creations for which I believe there is a *preferable image*. By design, we each possess exclusive physical characteristics, and there is a rendering of you that best mirrors this design. Identifying and pursuing that design, it would seem, would be a worthwhile goal for anyone.

Have you ever stopped to consider that there is a "best version of you"? I'm not talking about what our culture might demand, but what God's enduring intent was when you sprang from His creative genius? If you believe you are just a random bipod created solely to sustain the human species, I suppose an exercise like this would seem pointless. From that perspective, your goal is simply surviving and becoming whatever feels good to you. But if your experience and understanding convince you that you were created on purpose, it becomes critically relevant to consider not just what you believe and accomplish, but also your physical state— your *"image and likeness."*

It is a diabolical reality that most people are so ashamed or repulsed by their nakedness that they won't even look at themselves in a mirror. It's also sadly instructive that the vast majority of lovemaking in the Western world takes place in total darkness. [2] If God thought there was something wrong with our physical forms, He would have hidden them behind fig leaves and furs from the get-go. *Our problem is not that we make too much of our bodies, but that we make too much of ourselves.* Adam and Eve experienced this truth firsthand, and we've all been dealing with the tragic consequences ever since. God celebrated our bodies as a masterstroke of His creativity, but our willfulness took what was designed for God's glory and hijacked it for our own.

The Biggest Loser

Who was the "biggest loser" when Adam and Eve were created and received the mantle of the "very-good-image-and-likeness-of-God?" That may seem like a strange question, but there was another created being that would have taken our creation as usurpation of his grandeur and authority. Previous to God's presentation of Adam and Eve as the crown of His creation, Lucifer, or Satan, would have been considered the most glorious created being. His pride and rebellion caused him to lose his heavenly standing, but there's no doubt that he was previously something marvelous to behold. He alone was allowed to "walk on the stones of fire" in the heavenly realms (Ezekiel 28:14). As one who opposed everything God intended, you can imagine what disdain and jealousy Satan felt toward these new bearers of God's image. *From the beginning, one of Satan's primary goals has been to mar, degrade, and compromise our ability to rightly carry and radiate God's glory.*

He accomplished this by enticing Adam and Eve to become rebels as well, and it's interesting to note that he used food, lies, and our own pride to do it. The spiritual ramifications of the fall of man are numerous, and the physical damage was significant. Created to sustain life forever, the bodies of Adam and Eve became mortal. [3] Created to delight God and each other, they became acutely aware of their physical bodies, which led them to a previously unknown experience of shame and body consciousness. This self-obsession poisoned their relationship with God and each other (Genesis 3:8-24). Created to perform all the tasks and purposes God assigned; they became susceptible to disease and dysfunction.

Fast-forward several millennia, and it's apparent we're reeling from the fallout of this spiritual, relational, and physiological disaster—and much of the broken-ness is ultimately expressed in our physical bodies. *Satan's campaign to distort God's image and likeness continues, and we too often cooperate by debasing our bodies through neglect, abuse, and idolatry.* Our thoughts and actions continue to repeat the mistakes of Eden as we consciously or subconsciously replay the mantra *"It's my body and I'll do what I want to with it."* Take a glance across the landscape of disfigured, rearranged, skeletal, deconditioned, diseased, and obese people in our culture and it's clear this kind of thinking rules the day. Take a look at those in our churches and, sadly, they often give no point of comparison.

All people are "fearfully and wonderfully made." We all bear the image and likeness of God. We remain the crown and pinnacle of God's creative work. [4] Acknowledging that God is deeply concerned with our spiritual health and well-being, I believe God also has a preferable and "best" physical image of you that He desires to express His glory. He wants to extend His Kingdom through you! As long as we refuse to walk in this calling and trade it for a self-serving or self-aggrandizing substitute, we will limit our ability to physically "declare the glory of God" along with the rest of creation.

The obstacles to declaring God's glory are many. We cannot return to the perfec-tion and innocence of early Eden. Acknowledging God's original will and design, however, should serve to raise our standards and inspire our pursuit of being *Fit For The King.*

---

1. Only North American pets and animals raised for food are ever overweight. I think it's safe to assume that all animal prototypes were designed and created as a "perfect" example of their species—neither gaunt, mutilated, or overweight.

2. *Let's Turn The Light Off Dear!* By Allan Hall. Mail Online March 28, 2012.

3. Despite being under the curse of sin, the first generations of mankind lived for hundreds of years. It's interesting to note Isaiah indicates that in the millennial Kingdom (the thousand-year reign of Jesus on earth before the new Heaven and Earth are created) even those who die a premature death will live to be at least 150 years old (Isaiah 65:20-23).

4. The issue of birth defects—genetic and hormonal abnormalities that affect weight and appearance—should be addressed. All life is sacred and of equal value. Handicaps and genetic and hormonal abnormalities are not a manifestation of personal sin, but of man-kind's fallen condition and God's permissive will. People with handicaps or inherited conditions can equally glorify God in their bodies by pursuing a godly stewardship of their lives as they are able. None of the contents of this book are targeted toward people who are incapable of changing their physical condition (temporarily or permanently). Rather, it is designed to provide information, challenge, encouragement, and practical help to the vast majority of people who are fully capable of determining and progressing toward a balanced physical state.

PART FIVE

TRANSFORMATION

CHAPTER 14

THE END GAME

For I am confident of this very thing, that He who began a good work in you will perfect it until the day of Christ Jesus. Philippians 1:6 (NASB)

Afterlife

'Cause every day the world is made
A chance to change, but I feel the same
And I wonder why would I wait 'til I die to come alive?
I'm ready now, I'm not waiting for the afterlife

Words and Music by Jon Foreman/Tim Foreman
©2013 Publishing Shmublishing

Perhaps the most critical question every follower of Jesus needs to answer is, *"What have I been saved for?"* How we answer this vital question will set the trajectory of our Christian walk, inform our daily decisions, and animate the vision we possess for our lives. Our answer also has major ramifications for the perspective we have of our physical bodies and our motives for maintaining them.

For most people, the answer to the question above is *"Heaven."* According to those who asked this question of professing Christians, a majority said, *"God sent His son Jesus to die for me so that I could go to Heaven after I die."* In answering this way, we can't help but order our lives as if we've already attained God's goal for us and subsequently marginalize all that takes place between now and our passing. This response makes Heaven the goal of the Christ-follower instead of a wonderful benefit. An answer like this begets another question: *If God's goal is to get us to Heaven, why doesn't He just take us there at the time of our salvation? What purpose do our lives on earth serve if all He really desires is our presence with Him?*

We've spent four chapters seeking to *demolish* wrong thinking that hinders us from acting biblically in regard to our bodies. These beliefs hold us hostage to false assumptions about our value and consequently lower our expectations of the plans God has for us. We've just completed three chapters that laid a *foundation* on which to build a new understanding of our bodies. I want to begin Part Five defining what the Bible clearly reveals as God's goal for every child of His: *Transformation.*

Rather than being the end-point of our spiritual pilgrimage, our salvation is actually the starting line. This is where God begins to glorify Himself by displaying His transforming work in all aspects of our lives: our characters, works, motives, and bodies. Left to our own devices and darkened thinking, our goals and physical bodies would conform to the priorities and lusts of our culture, without regard for God's design, ownership, or purposes. Under His rule, we have the capacity and obligation to prove that Jesus does more than change our eternal destination; His Holy Spirit initiates a transformative work in our lives that continues until we attain Christlikeness when we enter God's presence.

What is God's Will For My Life?

An age-old question asked predominantly by those in their twenties is, "What is God's will for my life?" The circumstances that give rise to this question are typically the kind of life transitions that involve choosing college majors, entering post-college careers, and marriage. While I am not prepared to give you career or dating advice, I can state categorically that I know what God's "big picture" will is for your life. How can I possibly know that? I can know because God's overarching will is the same for all of our lives—continuous transformation into the likeness of Christ.

The Bible contains the blueprint for all who consider themselves a follower of Jesus.

"And we know that God causes all things to work together for good [1] to those who love God, to those who are called according to His purpose. For those whom He foreknew, He also predestined to become conformed to the image of His Son, so that He would be the firstborn among many brethren." Romans 8:28-29 (NASB)

While the new believer experiences a radical transformation of eternal destination—from death to life—changes to our characters, language, desires, and bodies happen over time, courtesy of the Holy Spirit and our cooperative obedience (1 Peter 1:14-16). Our transformation will be complete in Heaven, but until then we live out this process day to day, with slow, steady progress being the expected norm.

> *"For the Lord is the Spirit, and wherever the Spirit of the Lord is,*
> *there is freedom* [from the kind of lives we used to live].
> *So all of us who have had that veil removed can see and*
> *reflect the glory of the Lord. And the Lord—who is the Spirit—makes*
> *us more and more like him as we are changed into his glorious image."*
> 2 Corinthians 3:17-18 (NLT) [comment mine]

Conforming or Transforming?

Perhaps the most difficult and persistent battle of transformation takes place in our physical bodies. Given to pleasure and self-will, our bodies become a battleground from the beginning of our walk with Christ. When explaining how a life of submission and worship develops, the Apostle Paul sets his sights squarely on the physical dimension of our transformation.

> *And so, dear brothers and sisters, I plead with you to give your bodies*
> *to God because of all he has done for you. Let them be a living and*
> *holy sacrifice—the kind he will find acceptable. This is truly the way to*
> *worship him. Don't copy the behavior and customs of this world,*
> *but let God transform you into a new person by changing the way you*
> *think. Then you will learn to know God's will for you,*
> *which is good and pleasing and perfect.*
> Romans 12:1-2 (NLT)

Our bodies need transforming and disciplining, but this can only happen when our minds are renewed to see with clarity the stakes that are involved.

The Pattern Of The World

Let's step outside our own personal fitness situation to see the template of our culture. The majority of people in our part of the world conform to two extremes: many lead sedentary, pleasure-filled lives that lead to obesity and resultant health problems, while others lead self-focused, narcissistic lives. In contrast to those who conform to the culture, others lead lives animated by consistent transformation and growth toward Christlikeness, physically and spiritually. A Christian seeking to avoid the extremes of our culture will pursue a transformed mind, which provides the motivation for transformed actions. Christians are called to live in the Transformation Zone, as shown in this chart, avoiding the extremes of the left and right.

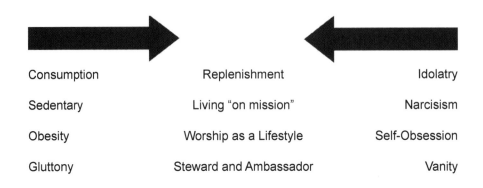

Consumption	Replenishment	Idolatry
Sedentary	Living "on mission"	Narcissism
Obesity	Worship as a Lifestyle	Self-Obsession
Gluttony	Steward and Ambassador	Vanity

TRANSFORMATION ZONE

Transformation Is Not An Option

"Healthy things grow" is an oft-used phrase of one of the pastors I serve with. The truth of this is readily seen in nature, businesses, and even the church. In contrast, stagnation or atrophy typifies things that are unhealthy, declining, or dying.

A recent vacation took our family to the Sequoia National Forest in central California. This amazing sanctuary is home to some of the oldest living things on earth. Towering up to 300 feet in height—the length of a football field—and thirty feet in diameter, sequoias grow for hundreds of years. Evidence of their longevity can be seen in a growth ring that each tree develops during each growing season. There is no such thing as a living sequoia that does not produce a new ring of growth around its circumference each year.

The same principle should be true of our lives. If we're not dead, we should be growing and transforming from conformity to culture into conformity with Christ's image; mirroring Him more closely with the passing of each year. If that's not happening, Scripture indicates something is interfering with a normative growth process.

We've all witnessed others on this journey from conformity to transformation to Christlikeness. The following are some common examples:

• The profane and irreverent individual who finds that his or her language is gradually transformed by the power of the Holy Spirit working in concert with their obedience in this area.

- The new believer who moves from ignorance and disinterest in Scripture to a hungry, inspired participant in regular Bible study.

- The family and marriage that is suffering from neglect and wrong priorities that becomes life-giving and vibrant when Christlike forgiveness is extended and biblical principles are practiced.

- The materialistic consumer who learns and practices God's principles for money, leading to contentment and proper financial stewardship.

Whatever the area of life and conduct, the life-changing power of the Holy Spirit coupled with our obedience produces observable results, always moving us to a greater ability to reflect Jesus.

What would you say to a professing believer whose language never changed years after his "conversion?" How about the individual who says she loves Jesus but remains disinterested in His Word, regular fellowship with other believers, or in giving to God's work? The Bible doesn't allow for authentic Christian lives without transformation. How we live our lives is the proof text that our relationship with God is genuine.

Since developing a biblical perspective of our physical bodies is the purpose of this volume, let's examine what transformation looks like in the area that the Apostle Paul identifies as the most reasonable place to look (Romans 12:1-2). Ask yourself these questions:

- Have I submitted my physical body to the Lord for His transformative work?

- Does my current physical state conform to the norms I see represented in the world or does it represent a life undergoing supernatural transformation?

- Do I look to the culture for cues as to my desired physical state or do I look to Scripture?

- Do I see the Fruits of the Spirit manifested and supported by my physical body?

Resources For A Daily Battle

Make no mistake, the unholy trinity of the world, the flesh, and the Devil set themselves against God's transformative work in our lives, and as I've described in earlier chapters, it's clear this war is currently raging in the Body of Christ. Jon Foreman of the band Switchfoot describes well the battle we enter when we engage this process of transformation.

Dare You To Move

Welcome to the fallout
Welcome to resistance
The tension is here
Tension is here
Between who you are and who you could be
Between how it is and how it should be
I dare you to move, I dare you to move
I dare you to lift yourself up off the floor
I dare you to move, I dare you to move
Like today never happened
Today never happened before.

Words and Music by Jon Foreman
© 2000 Meadowgreen Music/Sugar Pete Songs (Administered by EMI-
CMG Publishing)
Used by permission

If we were left to our own devices, and transformational success was simply a matter of "gutting it out" or "trying harder," we would be doomed to failure on every front. Thankfully, God hasn't set the high standard of imitating Jesus and then left us without resources to accomplish what He's called us to. God's very presence in the Holy Spirit ensures that we have all the resources necessary to see gradual transformation take place in all areas of our lives. As we've already read in 2 Corinthians 3, it is the Spirit who gives us the freedom from cultural conformity, old habits, and old ways of thinking, as well as the power to blaze new trails of transformational obedience in our bodies. Let's not sell short the presence of God's Spirit, even if this battle looms large in our lives. Paul reminds us of the power of the Holy Spirit.

But if the Spirit of Him who raised Jesus from the dead dwells in you, He who raised Christ Jesus from the dead will also give life to your mortal bodies through His Spirit who dwells in you. Romans 8:11 (NASB)

If the Holy Spirit possesses the power to raise a body from the dead (and don't we believe He will do this ultimately for each of us anyway?), surely He is capable of guiding us toward healthier lives and bodies that best reflect His likeness. Singer/ songwriter Tim Timmons speaks about our tendency to underestimate God's power to transform in his song.

Christ In Me

The same great light that broke the dark
The same great peace that calmed the seas
Hallelujah, is living in me
The same great love that gives us breath
The same great power that conquered death
Hallelujah, is flowing through me
And what, what if I believed in Your power
And I really lived it
What, what if I believed Christ in me
What if I believed?
I would lay my worries down
See these hills as level ground
What if I believed, Christ in me
Oh, I would praise You with my life
Let my story lift you high
What if I believed, Christ in me?

Words and Music By Tim Timmons
© Letsbebeautiful/Sony/ATV Cross Keys Publishing, Sony/ATV Timber
Publishing/West Main Music
Used by permission

Transformative living is not for the faint of heart, so it's comforting to know that we've been called into this new way of living by a gracious and loving God Who promises to work with us to accomplish His purposes of complete transformation. *What's necessary from us is surrender to both the process and the enabler of the process—the Holy Spirit.* If you haven't done that, now would be a great time. This is one of those prayers God always answers in the affirmative because it's in keeping with His expressed will for all His children:

Dear Jesus, I am convinced from Scripture that You desire transformation in all aspects of my life. I confess that out of ignorance of my calling or disobedience I have hindered the work Your Holy Spirit is seeking to accomplish in my mind, body, and spirit. Understanding Your will for my life is continuous transformation, I surrender my mind and body to you and ask for the Spirit's strength, direction, and inspiration as I journey toward greater obedience in my life. Help me in every way to cooperate in the work of transformation You are seeking to accomplish. I claim the promise of Ephesians 3:20-21 that as I continue to surrender to Your work, You will do 'exceedingly, abundantly, beyond what I can ask or think' for Your glory according to the Power that works within me. Amen.

More biblical encouragement for this journey of transformation is ahead, along with practical steps from Joe that will give you the tools necessary to see it to completion. I leave you for now with the same benediction the Apostle Paul gave to the ancient church at Thessalonica in Greece as they pursued the goal of Christ-likeness.

Now may the God of peace Himself sanctify you entirely; and may your spirit and soul and body be preserved complete, without blame at the coming of our Lord Jesus Christ. Faithful is He who calls you, and He also will bring it to pass. 1 Thessalonians 5:23-24 (NASB)

---

1.   Note that the "good" that transpires here is not some serendipitous outcome from a bad situation, but a transformation in our character (often through difficult circumstances) to better reflect Jesus.

CHAPTER 15

HIDING IN PLAIN SIGHT
(NUTRITION PART 1)

Like most rural Iowa families, mine planted a vegetable garden in our expansive backyard each spring. Tomato, pepper, radish, carrot, and squash seeds were pressed into the dark soil, watering cans were enlisted, and seed packet markers were erected on popsicle sticks a couple of weeks after the last of the winter frost was out of the ground. Optimism for summer and fall harvests abounded each new season as dirt ground its way under our fingernails and into the knees of our jeans. But our optimism often vanished as we faced sober reality when scrawny root vegetables were unearthed in June. This sad reality turned to public shame when undersized peppers, tomatoes, and squash were carried to the house in July and August. It seemed that no matter how much the Tewells watered, weeded, or hoped for horticultural success, our garden never reached its potential.

Adding to our frustration and embarrassment was the bumper crop of vegetables harvested by our backyard neighbors, the Kennedys. Although both family garden plots experienced identical amounts of sunlight, rainfall, extra watering, and sweat, the Kennedy vegetables were larger, more colorful, and more numerous than ours.

Curious as to the secret of their success, I began spying on them whenever I saw them working in their garden. Peeking between the slats of the fence separating our yards, I learned of critical differences in their gardening practices that resulted in such healthy end products. Before they planted each spring, they incorporated a large pile of steer manure into their plot, fortifying the soil. Additionally, they watered with a sprayer that dispensed a nutrient-rich liquid fertilizer onto the maturing plants several times each season. As if that potent combination wasn't enough, they also used insecticides that kept aphids and other pests from leaching production capacity from the plants.

Important lessons can be learned from these two garden plots: The superior nutrition and protection provided by the Kennedys made all the difference when harvest time arrived. While we were withholding nutrition and protection from our plants, our neighbors were unlocking the full potential of their garden through proper feeding and care.

The Priority of Proper Nutrition

Similar to the two gardens in my story, your physical health is more impacted by what you provide your body through proper nutrition than by your fitness goals, how much time you spend exercising, or the quality of the equipment you use. I filled my gyms with the latest equipment so committed members could work themselves into a lather several times per week. Still, many of these people were nutritionally deficient, making little or no progress in their quest for physical health. At the same time, there were members who were nutritionally compliant and enjoyed excellent health with much less time spent in vigorous exercise.

When a client meets with me at a gym, I provide significant guidance for their workout regimens. I spend a great deal of time with them, reviewing their nutritional logs (I call them "habit-trackers"), performing body-composition analysis, and constructing meal plans. I provide a nutritional emphasis because I'm well aware that a week of intense training can be undermined by a weekend of poor food choices.

For most people in the world, dinner consists of choosing between a limited number of staple foods, most of which are naturally derived and nutritionally dense. In America, we are blessed and burdened with broad food choices, which necessitate discernment. Unlike most of the planet, we are not shopping at the farmer's market but are pushing a large cart through air-conditioned aisles bursting with man-made, preserved, packaged, and shelf-stable offerings designed for convenience. Many of these highly processed options claim to contain "healthy" ingredients. How do we learn to make wise choices? How can we outsmart multinational food corporations with all their marketing savvy? What does it mean that a food is "natural," "vitamin-fortified," "whole grain," or "organic?" Are "lite," "fat-free," or "sugar-free" offerings really better for you, particularly if they are loaded with stabilizers and flavor enhancers?

As I joined my wife on a trip to the grocery store this week, I was sobered and distressed to again witness the abundance of nutritionally vacant foods that enjoyed eye-level placement, end-of-aisle displays, and fire-sale prices. While healthy food options are growing, I was reminded that this battle is still in its infancy.

It's a battle that is being waged when we gather as the Church in our various meeting places during the week, as well. A review of the Sunday morning food and beverage available at my church includes cookies, crackers, bagels, donuts, coffee, and lemonade, in addition to two popular soda machines. Just recently, we accepted a donated vending machine that is now dispensing a colorful variety of sugar, fat, and oil-laden convenience foods. But the profits go to our Missions work! With offerings like this, it's hard to escape the message that is being communicated to our congregation.

Hiding In Plain Sight

Despite the potential for confusion, most people already possess the information they need to make a transformation in their nutritional health. When I ask new clients to name foods that will allow their health to flourish, there's no hesitation in their responses: "Fresh fruits and vegetables, whole grains, and lean meats." When asked to name foods that erode health, sheepish grins precede responses such as, "Fast food, sweets, and soda." When I explain the need to do the majority of shopping around the perimeter areas of the grocery store, I receive nods of recognition. People already know much of the truth regarding food and health, but like Adam and Eve in the Garden, even one poor alternative is too many for us to turn down. Imagine how quickly The Fall would have happened if God had created more than one tree of forbidden fruit!

Evolution Of A Nutritional Crisis

A myriad of health issues have emerged in our country over the past forty years. It's also true that exercise was not a main factor in our nation's better health profile until deep into the 1900s. Then came the 1970's and an explosion of frozen-food products such as TV dinners, which grocery stores accommodated through expanded freezer space. Food processing, formerly a mostly localized industry, increasingly took place far away from the end consumer, which resulted in a greater use of preservatives. Other significant factors impacting the way we eat have been the rise of the two-income household, the introduction of the microwave oven, and, ironically, the proliferation of youth sports. Youth sports and working moms have kept kids and parents busy in early evening when meal prep takes place. Grocery stores that offered a meat counter, vegetables, fruit, dairy, and some canned and boxed staples began to change with the times. They expanded their shelf space to accept thousands of new products designed to make meal preparation fast and easy for the beleaguered mother and wife (and hungry kids).

Breakfast that used to consist of oatmeal, wheat bread toast, eggs, bacon, shredded wheat, milk, orange juice, and fresh fruit morphed into on-the-go breakfast. The new breakfast consisted of toaster-baked pastries, sugar-laden cereals, and sugary orange drinks. The fast-food drive-thru got busy, too, offering egg sandwiches, greasy hash browns, donuts, and other high-calories items that can be wolfed down on the way to school.

Lunch changed too. The new standards are deep-fried chicken nuggets, pudding cups, potato chips, sodas, oversized burritos, and sixteen-inch submarine sandwiches.

Dinner that included meat, pasta, fresh vegetables, rice, beans and milk was largely replaced by take-out pizza and burgers, microwaved entrées, and a variety of "just add water" boxed mixes. To top it off, have the obligatory dessert. You don't want to read the nutrition-facts labeling.

Our transformation from a homemade-meal society to a convenience-food society has been very detrimental to our national health. It seems ironic that our cable channels are filled with cooking shows featuring made-from-scratch meals, while the vast majority of Americans are "assembling" meals or heading to the drive-thru on the way home from work. A quarter of our population eats dinner as a family less than three nights per week,[1] and for those that do eat together the average time spent at the dinner table has shrunk from over an hour to twelve minutes. [2] It's not a stretch to say that convenience is killing us, and the true cost of this sea change in diet is staggering. All the same foods that sustained us for centuries are available in our modern behemoth marketplaces; they are just lost in the mind-numbing array of other products that are squeezing them off the shelves.

Getting back on track by eating nutritious meals is one of the great challenges most will have in becoming *Fit For The King*. There is no question that this will involve daily, countercultural decisions based on the conviction that we owe it to God and ourselves to maintain our bodies as He intended. It's really not difficult. Nutrition comes from real food, not just a multivitamin. We need only consume the calories that we need to survive, and these are available in abundance.

So what is so difficult about this approach to eating? Here you have to be honest. Are you willing to take the time to source nutritionally sound foods that will provide your body and mind what it needs to grow stronger, heal, and think clearly?

Pick up a rotisserie chicken, instead of a pizza. Select a fast food outlet with fresh vegetable and lean meat options (skip the chips, sodas, and cookies). Open up a recipe book or go online for some of your favorite celebrity chef offerings. Plan the meals you and your family will eat. Make a list of the staples and ingredients you need before you go grocery shopping—and stick to it. Shop the perimeter of the store, avoiding most of the freezer aisle, the snack aisle, the pop aisle, and the boxed baking mixes (nearly everything that offers a coupon in the Sunday paper). If you have kids, they will undoubtedly complain if you cut back on the treats and soda, but somebody's got to be the adult and get this nutrition issue turned around.

If you really want to impress, start your own vegetable garden. But don't forget the manure and nutrient-rich liquid fertilizer.

1. *Empty Seats: Fewer Families Eat Together.* By Heather Mason Kiefer, January 20, 2004. *www.gallup.com.*
2. *Family Dinner Challenge.* The Six O'Clock Scramble, *www.thescramble.com.*

CHAPTER 16

THE BRAND NEW YOU
(THE END OF THE ZOMBIE APOCALYPSE)

If we in our own strength confide
Our striving would be losing
—Martin Luther

In January 2014 one of the most bizarre life stories of World War 2 came to an end. Hiroo Onoda, a Japanese intelligence officer trained in guerilla warfare and deployed in 1944 to the Philippine island of Lubang, died at the age of ninety-one in Tokyo. Onoda became famous when he was discovered in 1974 still fighting a war he believed had persisted for twenty-seven years after it officially ended. Despite leaflet drops, Japanese military communications, newspaper drops, and even a personal visit from a Japanese compatriot, Onoda kept up his harassment of Philippine villagers from his jungle hideout. He was convinced that all entreaties to surrender were a ruse of the enemy to flush him out and capture him. Only after a visit from a Japanese army major did Onoda finally realize that he'd spent all those years fighting a war that was officially over. Recalling the day that reality finally hit home, Onoda wrote:

"Suddenly everything went black. A storm raged inside me. I felt like a fool for having been so tense and cautious on the way here [to surrender]. Worse than that, what had I been doing for all these years? ... I eased off the pack that I always carried with me and laid the gun on top of it. Would I really have no more use for this rifle that I had polished and cared for like a baby all these years .... Had the war really ended thirty years ago?" [1]

Ignorance often carries a high price. Hiroo Onoda and the many he had needlessly killed, injured, and robbed for nearly three decades all paid a high price because of his ignorance and disbelief. Financially, vocationally, relationally, physically, and spiritually, we all have experienced the truths of this verse:

"My people are destroyed for lack of knowledge." Hosea 4:6 (NASB)

The High Price of Ignorance

My ignorance of leadership and management agendas has cost me years of vocational and ministerial frustration in past positions. If I had only known what I was getting myself into, I could have invested my efforts in more fruitful endeavors. All of us have experienced interpersonal friction with family, friends, and spouses that, due to our ignorance, resulted in stepping on emotional minefields we didn't know existed. In the area of health and fitness, skipped medical exams, sedentary lifestyles, and blissful ignorance of the nutritional deficiencies of our diets lead to rude awakenings when deferred care finally brings us to the doctor's office.

Ignorance of spiritual truths is of great consequence as well, and lead to unneeded struggles, barriers, and defeat in many areas of our lives, including the physical. Joe and I are continually hearing about the frustration Christ-followers are experiencing in their quest to change their fitness and nutritional habits. The barriers to lasting change could be summarized: "Try as I might, I just can't seem to change the destructive patterns and poor eating habits of my life." It's quite possible that you can relate to this statement, and perhaps in a moment of honest introspection you've brought yourself to utter similar words.

Spiritual Ignorance With Physical Repercussions

We learned in Chapter 14 that transformation—not Heaven—is the goal of a Christ-follower. But where physical transformation may be needed, we often encounter numerous detours and exit ramps that hinder and derail our cooperation with the Holy Spirit. In the same way that Old Testament characters were continually frustrated by their inability to follow The Law, we also often find ourselves incapable of making the progress toward God-honoring body care that we know God desires. New Year's resolutions, "trying harder," "gutting it out," and seeking inspiration from any and all sources becomes a vicious cycle that inevitably ends in failure. We relate to the Apostle Paul when he laments that he needs to be "saved from this body of death" due to his inability to consistently have victory over his fleshly desires (Romans 7:24). If you can relate to Paul's exasperation and have had a history of failure in your attempts to align your lifestyle with Scripture, God's Word has good news for you. As a Christian, the weak-willed, failure-prone, and self-gratifying person you once were is already dead. Also dead and buried is the narcissistic, self-absorbed, attention-starved, mirror-gazing, stage-seeking devotee of the superficial.

Boxing With Spiritual Shadows

Similar to the way we once feared imaginary monsters under our childhood beds, most followers of Christ surrender power and control to their old nature (a life outside of Christ that does not seek to please God or obey His word), even though it has been slain and rendered powerless. Many of us cower under the covers of well-worn habits and comfortable routines, seeking protection from and victory over lifestyle zombies that don't exist.

Paul makes a wonderful statement of hope and rebirth.

Therefore if anyone is in Christ, he is a new creature; the old things passed away; behold, new things have come. 2 Corinthians 5:17 (NASB)

The "old things" that are dead (passed away) are the desires and activities of our old nature, that part of us that was entirely resistant to God, was completely self-willed, and was unwilling and unable to obey and please Him. Our old nature was what caused us to be "slaves of sin" (Romans 6:6), unable to make righteous choices. We were condemned to spiritually and physically destructive routines until, by God's grace, the Holy Spirit awoke in us the possibility that there was a whole other way of doing life—one that embraced the freedom made possible by Jesus' saving work on the cross.

All Things Made New

One of the "new things" that has come to those in Christ is the new nature we have received courtesy of our standing in Jesus. This is, literally and practically, a "brand new you" with a new eternal residency (New Heaven and Earth), a new moral compass (Holy Spirit), a new nature (with new motives and a desire to please God), a new purpose (glorifying God), and a new life goal (transformation). These are all things that are impossible for us to achieve, but God, in His sovereign power and undeserved grace, included all these incredible benefits and "upgrades" at the moment we came to saving faith in Jesus.

We are helpless to save ourselves, and we are equally helpless to empower the transformation God begins to make in our physical and spiritual lives. The practical mechanics of how we appropriate the power of this new nature are outlined in the New Testament books of Galatians and Romans. Both passages underscore the necessity that we die to ourselves before Jesus' new life can be lived out through us.

> *I have been crucified with Christ; and it is no longer I who live, but*
> *Christ lives in me; and the life which I now live in the flesh I live by faith*
> *in the Son of God, who loved me and gave Himself up for me.*
> *Galatians 2:20 (NASB)*

Paul gives more detail about our union with Christ—in both His death and resurrection:

> *Well then, should we keep on sinning so that God can show us more and more*
> *of his wonderful grace? Of course not! Since we have died to sin, how can we*
> *continue to live in it? Or have you forgotten that when we were joined with Christ*
> *Jesus in baptism, we joined him in his death? For we died and were buried with*
> *Christ by baptism. [2] And just as Christ was raised from the dead by the glorious*
> *power of the Father, now we also may live new lives.*
> *Since we have been united with him in his death, we will also be raised to life as he*
> *was. We know that our old sinful selves were crucified with Christ so that sin might*
> *lose its power in our lives. We are no longer slaves to sin. For when we died with*
> *Christ we were set free from the power of sin ... do not let sin control the way you*
> *live, do not give in to sinful desires. Do not let any part of your body become an*
> *instrument of evil to serve sin. Instead, give yourselves completely to God, for you*
> *were dead, but now you have new life. So use your whole body as an instrument*
> *to do what is right for the glory of God. Sin is no longer your master, for you no*
> *longer live under the requirements of the law. Instead, you live under the freedom*
> *of God's grace. Romans 6:1-7;12-14 (NLT)*

New Nature Has Replaced The Old Nature

Paul admonishes us to live free from the control of sin and to glorify God with our bodies. This would be a heavy burden if we were left to our own ability to do battle with an old nature that was still active and formidable. In fact, it would be downright unfair for him to tell us to do something that was next to impossible. He can boldly call us to this kind of liberated life, however, because our old nature is a vanquished foe, replaced by a new nature, which wants to please and obey God. When we understand and act on the fact that our old, unresponsive, and unwilling nature is dead and gone courtesy of our "baptism into Christ's death," we are liberated to a lifestyle marked more by spiritual victories than defeats.

If we have truly died to ourselves and entered into a new life empowered by Christ, our old nature is not a zombie that continually rises back from the dead to vex our progress toward transformation. In the book of Colossians, the Apostle Paul again addresses our sinful nature by reminding us that our slavery to a formerly dominant sinful bent has been both circumcised (surgically removed) and crucified (nailed to Jesus' cross). In the second chapter of his letter, Paul writes:

> *When you came to Christ, you were 'circumcised', but not by a physical procedure. Christ performed a spiritual circumcision—the cutting away of your sinful nature. For you were buried with Christ when you were baptized. And with Him you were raised to new life because you trusted the mighty power of God, who raised Christ from the dead. You were dead because of your sins and because your sinful nature was not yet cut away. Then God made you alive with Christ, for He forgave all our sins. He canceled the record of the charges against us and took it away by nailing it to the cross. In this way, He disarmed the spiritual rulers and authorities. He shamed them publicly by His victory over them on the cross. ... You have died with Christ, and He has set you free from the spiritual powers of this world. Colossians 2:11-15, 20 (NLT)*

Paul uses these words to identify our old nature: "cut away," "buried," "forgiven," "cancelled," "took away and nailed to the cross," "disarmed," "shamed publically," "dead." Clearly, our old nature is in no position to influence us any longer.

Instead, courtesy of Christ's work on the cross and the Holy Spirit's presence in our lives, Paul uses these words to describe us as we are now: "raised to new life," "alive with Christ," "forgiven," "victory," "set free."

Spiritual Truth Becomes Practical Reality

A question routinely arises among believers from this statement of fact regarding the death of the old nature:

"How is it, if my old nature is dead, I still struggle daily with the various aspects of the transformation God is seeking to work in me? Why do I always fail in my attempts to establish consistent patterns of God-honoring body care?"

This is a reality we all live in. We need to understand that one of the forces we're doing battle with—too often in our own efforts—is the unrelenting foe of our flesh. Our ignorance of the superiority of Christ's power keeps far too many "on the ropes," spiritually speaking, when He wants us to be champions.

What all followers of Christ (including Paul) deal with daily is the unholy trio of the world, the flesh, and the Devil. "The World" is the ungodly system and culture we all live in. We can expect it to consistently give us the wrong rationales, motives, goals, and desires because it is fallen, unredeemed, and not looking for godly solutions. The world tells us we "only live once" and should do all we can to maximize our enjoyment of life. It suggests that "if it feels good, do it" and that there will never be negative consequences for our actions. It proclaims that your body is "your business" and "belongs to you." Some of the world's messages are obviously false, but most are skillfully nuanced and are usually designed to bring immediate gratification. We are called to be discerning and we must sift what we hear from our culture through the filter of Scripture to see if it aligns with God's revealed truth. While we can choose to follow cultural thinking and actions to do right or wrong, this is done of our own free will— the world does not hold power over us to force us to misbehave (Romans 12:2, 1 Corinthians 1:20, Philippians 2:15, Colossians 2:8, 1 John 2:15–16).

"The Devil" represents the unseen but powerful spiritual forces at work around us. While our battle to consistently pursue healthy habits may feel like a 12-rounder with Lucifer himself, it is doubtful any of us commands the attention of Satan (who is not omnipresent). Nonetheless, Paul reminds us that these forces are real, are doing battle in a parallel dimension, and are often the ones influencing those who oppose God's Kingdom (Ephesians 6:12). We do not need to fear their power and they cannot make us behave in ways we do not choose (1 John 4:2-4). God has provided spiritual armor that repels the weapons of the spiritual world (Ephesians 6:10–17).

Our flesh, on the other hand, is a formidable foe that even Paul found a hindrance in his pursuit of godly living.

> *For I know that nothing good dwells in me, that is, in my flesh; for the willing is present in me, but the doing of the good is not. For the good that I want, I do not do, but I practice the very evil that I do not want.*
> *Romans 7:18-19 (NASB)*

The new nature possessed by believers can obey and please God, and has the desire to do so. This nature does battle daily against the flesh—the remnant of our physical ties to Adam that still exercises self-will. While I don't want to understate the power of our flesh, it is imperative we understand that as Sprit-filled creatures possessing new natures, we clearly have the upper hand. If we consistently cave in to our fleshly desires, this would indicate our lives need focused prayer, spiritual discipline, and greater accountability. At some points in life, we must remember and understand where we stand with the Lord. God knows our flesh will be a constant source of wrong thinking and bad ideas, so He warns us not to let our guards down and to appropriate the fullness of the Spirit as we do battle:

But put on the Lord Jesus Christ, and make no provision
for the flesh in regard to its lusts.
Romans 13:14 (NASB)

But I say, walk by the Spirit, and you will not carry out the desire of the
flesh. For the flesh sets its desire against the Spirit, and the Spirit against
the flesh; for these are in opposition to one another,
so that you may not do the things that you please.
Galatians 5:16-17 (NASB)

It's interesting to note that in the passage above the things "you please" (what you would like to do) are the naturally God-pleasing inclinations—not sinful ones—that arise from your new nature that desires to please the Lord.

Walking in Consistent Victory

So what is the real culprit behind our persistent failure to experience transformation in our physical bodies? Since the power of our old nature has been cancelled by our union with Jesus, and we hold the upper hand in the ongoing battle with the world, the Devil, and our flesh, we should be celebrating victory over sin every day.

Several responses seem plausible:

1. We desire to be faithful in the area of body stewardship but have
   been living in ignorance of the reality of our victory over our old
   nature. Many of us also ignore the resources at our disposal for
   gaining victory over our remaining foes.

2. We have never viewed properly maintaining our bodies as a
   discipleship or maturity issue.

3. We agree this is a problem area for us, but have never felt convicted that change was necessary.

To those who relate to response #1, you now have God's truth that can be brought to bear in your personal journey. Memorize, personalize, and internalize the Scriptures I've cited to encourage you in your physical transformation. Follow through on the prescriptions Joe will be presenting in his chapters on proper nutrition and exercise.

For those who favor response #2, I hope that this book has brought you to the point of understanding that how we care for our bodies is of great importance to

God and is a central part of what it means to grow in our likeness of Christ.

For those identifying with response #3, I hope you will continue to read the upcoming chapters with an open heart and mind. Ask the Holy Spirit to bring whatever conviction might be necessary and be willing, in His power, to make any changes He provokes. If you honestly don't possess a desire to please and obey God and feel no real conviction regarding lifestyle issues that are contrary to Scripture, it's quite likely you're still operating under the old nature. You simply don't possess the new nature that comes when one places their faith in Jesus.

Believing The Transformed Life Is The Best Life

I would like to suggest one other possibility that might get to the root of our inability or unwillingness to change our behavior: Perhaps we're not yet convinced that God's love for us is perfect, that His ways are always superior, and that Jesus is better than what the world offers. Despite what we have been told in Scripture (and what we would likely say if asked), a voice in our head tells us that we will be missing out on something great if we completely surrender to God's ownership of our bodies and Jesus' lordship over our lives. A belief that God is holding out on us is as old as original sin. This deeply false belief is the seedbed in which most of our disobedience takes root.

No matter the arena of our struggle, may we all become convinced that transformation into the likeness of Christ is God's purpose for each of us, that the resources He has given us are sufficient to do the job, and that His unfathomable love for us is what motivates His commands.

The Apostle Paul, who has informed most of the teaching in this chapter, is overcome with emotion as he describes all that is available to us as we press on toward the goal of transformation.

> *When I think of all this, I fall to my knees and pray to the Father, the Creator of everything in heaven and on earth. I pray that from his glorious, unlimited resources he will empower you with inner strength through his Spirit. Then Christ will make his home in your hearts as you trust in him. Your roots will grow down into God's love and keep you strong. And may you have the power to understand, as all God's people should, how wide, how long, how high, and how deep his love is. May you experience the love of Christ, though it is too great to understand fully. Then you will be made complete with all the fullness of life and power that comes from God. Now all glory to God, who is able, through his mighty power at work within us, to accomplish infinitely more than we might ask or think. Ephesians 3:14-20 (NLT)*

It's clear from this passage that a conviction regarding God's love is a prime motivator of our behavior. Trusting in the authenticity of His love causes us to "put down roots" and gives us the stability and strength to turn a deaf ear to the siren song of the world, the Devil, and our own flesh when it cries out for gratification.

If, like Hiroo Onoda, you've spent years fighting wars that were spiritually over and settled long ago, may you now walk with new confidence marked by victory! God sees a brand new you, who is not dictated by past failures, the opinions of others, or even by what you think of yourself. Out of all the "better candidates" in the world, He's chosen to make you an object of His love, mercy, and glory. Return His loving embrace. Walk with Him in loving obedience. Become a vessel through which He can accomplish great things for His glory alone.

I Am New

Now I won't deny
The worst you could say about me
But I'm not defined by mistakes that I've made
Because God says of me
I am not who I was
I am being remade
I am new
I am chosen and holy and I'm dearly loved
I am new
Too long I have lived in the shadows of shame
Believing that there was no way I could change
But the One who is making everything new
Doesn't see me the way that I do…
I am not who I was
I am being remade
I am new
I am chosen and holy and I'm dearly loved
I am new
Dead to the old man, I'm coming alive I am new
Forgiven, beloved, hidden in Christ
Made in the image of the Giver of Life
Righteous and holy, reborn and remade
Accepted and worthy, this is our new name
This is who we are now

Words and Music by Jason Gray and Joel Hanson
© 2009 Centricity Music Publishing/Where's Rocky Music
Used by permission

1. No Surrender: My Thirty Year War by Hiroo Onoda. BlueJacket Books, 1974.
2. The baptism referred to here is not physical baptism per se, but the union we experience spiritually with Christ in His death and resurrection.

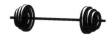

CHAPTER 17

THRIVING VERSUS SURVIVING (NUTRITION PART 2)

Thrive

Been fighting things that I can't see
Like voices coming from the inside of me and
Like doing things I find hard to believe in
Am I myself or am I dreaming?
I've been awake for an hour or so
Checking for a pulse but I just don't know
Am I a man when I feel like a ghost?
The stranger in the mirror is wearing my clothes
No, I'm not alright
I know that I'm not right
A steering wheel don't mean you can drive
A warm body don't mean I'm alive
No, I'm not alright
I know that I'm not right
Feel like I travel but I never arrive
I wanna thrive not just survive

Words and Music by Jon Foreman/ Publishing Shmublishing

August is approaching as I write this chapter, and in Iowa that means it's time for the Iowa State Fair. This annual extravaganza celebrating all things horticultural attracts over one million people each year from a state with a population of just two million. The fair inspired a Broadway musical and a subsequent movie, and this popular attraction is a study in contrasts. The city residents, dressed in shorts and loafers, are shoulder-to-shoulder on the Grand Concourse with the farmers and ranchers in their Stetson hats and cowboy boots. Small town cloggers and square dancers share the stage with hog callers and 1970s hair bands.

The main attraction for many, however, is the fair food; and it's among the belly-bursting gauntlet of food vendors that we find the most confusing array of mixed messages. The same National Turkey Federation that touts the nutritional benefits of lean poultry sells thousands of turkey legs as a single-course meal containing 1,136 calories. The Iowa Cattlemen's Association promotes their protein and iron-rich products, while cashing in on a 710-calorie beef sundae, and the Iowa Pork Congress reminds us that their white-meat chops are best consumed as a 736-calorie pork chop on a stick. Across from the impressive display of vegetables in the Agriculture Building are food wagons selling deep-fried candy bars and cream-filled pastries (about 450 calories each), and quart-size buckets full of chocolate chip cookies. Tucked somewhere off the beaten path is a vendor selling fresh-cut fruit, and I think I remember seeing a skewer of reasonably nutritious grilled chicken and vegetables once—but I wouldn't swear to it.

There is another vendor that's opened for business at the entrance gates the past couple of years in response to large demand: mobility scooters. The fairgrounds are now covered with these and I'm wondering how many people have made the connection between what we're consuming and the apparent inability of a surprising percentage of our population to walk more than a few minutes at a time.

I'll acknowledge that you don't go to the state fair expecting to find the same food offerings as at a health fair, but in many ways what you experience at the fair is a microcosm of the choices you must make every day. You are literally deluged with food and beverage options daring you to make wise choices. More often than not, making a nutritious choice is like finding a needle in a haystack.

I'm not going to patronize you with a detailed list of "best" food choices beyond what David and I listed as our core foods in Chapter Twelve. Nearly everybody understands product labels and Surgeon General warnings. You know what foods are intrinsically "good" for us and "bad" for us. You know that if you're choosing to create a dinner by adding water to something that's shelf stable, preserved, loaded with salt and sugar, and in a box, you've already made a number of nutritional compromises. Ditto most offerings at fast-food restaurants. If you accept the fact that our nutritional deficiencies are not a product of ignorance, you have to look elsewhere to discover why you consistently make poor choices that sabotage your health.

Instead, I'm going to present six cultural and personal issues you must confront if you're going to find success in providing your body what it needs to thrive. Rather than provide a list of foods you must consume or avoid, I'd rather cut to the heart of what's keeping you nutritionally deprived and physically unfit.

I call them the *Six A's of the Nutritional Apocalypse: Available, Acquired, Appropriate, Affordable, Acceptable, Acute.*

Available Time

Given the large amount of modern devices created to increase efficiency, it would be reasonable to expect that this generation possesses vast quantities of disposable time. Ironically, nothing could be further from the truth. Whether meaningful or mindless, something always rushes in to fill any free moment you have. Good nutrition takes time, whether it's planning a week's worth of meals, making a nutritionally superior lunch, or cooking some basic foods in advance to use later. When good nutrition becomes important to you, you'll sacrifice time in front of the TV or computer screen to fix a proper dinner. Or you'll enlist the help of a spouse or family member to do chores, which frees you up to create a meal that will support your commitment to good health.

Sadly, our health doesn't often become a priority to us until we face a crisis that causes us to re-evaluate our schedules or lifestyles. We reap what we sow and the sudden nature of payback is devastating. God instituted a principle for us when He ordered His week to include a day of rest. It follows that we need quiet day in our own weeks. Along with time to reflect on God's goodness and instruction for your life, what could be more important than using some of your day of rest to plan a healthy, nutritionally balanced menu for the week ahead?

Typically, Sunday evenings are when my wife and I grill chicken breasts or cook brown rice to use later in the week. Instead of reaching for a packaged or frozen meal some night, we have better options because of our preplanning.

Acquired Taste

We have become accustomed to levels of salt and sugar in our food that previous generations would have found inedible. At times it seems as if the food is simply a vehicle for delivering salt and sugar to our bodies. Seasonings and condiments operate under a law of diminishing returns. You'll probably enjoy your meat or vegetables just as much if you cut your toppings and additives in half. By impulsively drenching our food with enhancers, the taste buds and the reward centers of our brains are literally being rewired to demand unhealthy levels of these ingredients.

It is possible, however, to detox your body and enjoy lower levels of seasoning and sweetness. If you add salt or sugar to your food after it's prepared, cut back. Make meals at home with less salt and sugar. When dining out, ask your server to reduce the sodium and/or MSG in your meal. Make more things at home versus buying them. Buy foods labeled "reduced sugar" or "lower sodium." Use fresh vegetables and fruits, instead of canned. Experiment with herbs and spices to add flavor, rather than relying on the saltshaker and sugar-laden condiments.

Use sweeteners such as agave nectar or stevia in your coffee, tea, and recipes, as an alternative to refined sugar. *See our website for condiment and seasoning alternatives.*

Appropriate Quantity

Take a trip to a restaurant overseas and you'll experience "portion shock." Compared to other countries, the quantity of food served at most U.S. restaurants is borderline embarrassing. Oversized buns, massive potatoes drowning in butter, sour cream, marshmallows, cinnamon sugar, heaping baskets of biscuits and bread (hundreds of largely empty calories that are consumed before the meal is even ordered), and the obligatory mass of french fries compete with half-pound beef patties and pork tenderloins covering every square inch of your oversized platter. Sadly, despite the quantity of food served, the nutritional quality is often quite poor. The average sit-down chain-restaurant meal contains twice the calories of a typical home-cooked alternative, along with 151 percent of recommended daily salt intake, 89 percent of daily fat and 60 percent of daily cholesterol. All this is accompanied by beverages, appetizers, and dessert. It's likely that a single fast food meal will meet your entire day's caloric needs, and breakfast is often the worst offender. Appetizers are another culprit. A single order may contain over 3,000 calories.

Then there's the slippery slope of "value pricing" that has become institutional-ized at many restaurants. Moving you up to a larger size or an extra side item when you hear "for only fifty cents more," it sounds like a bargain until you realize it's far more food than you need. Another version growing in popularity is the "pack-age deal," where an appetizer, entrée, and dessert are "all included for just twenty dollars." You typically wouldn't order an appetizer or dessert but this deal is too good to pass up!

You already know this ... right? So split your meals with someone else. Avoid the trap of ordering a "bargain" that is more than you really want to eat. At a restaurant, ask for a to-go box to be brought out with your meal, then put half of the food in the container before you eat. Your server might even do this before bringing your food to the table, if you ask nicely. Patronize restaurants where the emphasis is on fresh, quality ingredients, rather than sheer quantity. Request vegetable substitutions to avoid the default of starchy, deep-fried side items. Restaurant chains large enough to be required to post calorie counts are typically serving food with 20 percent fewer calories than smaller chains or independent restaurants that are not required to publicize calorie content. [1] The point here is that most restaurants will offer healthier choices if they are required to disclose calorie content and nutritional information.

Affordable Convenience

Humans have been seeking ways to make life more convenient since Abel's first sacrifice. While many modern conveniences have the benefit of actually making our lives safer and healthier (think refrigerators, adhesive bandages, and blood glucose test strips), healthy food and convenience meals are often non sequiturs. These packaged foods are only designed to be fast and cheap.

Food chemistry and engineering make it possible to flake, form, and transport food products that are widely accessible, inexpensive, and pleasing to the palate. While these don't have to be budget busters, eating nutritionally sound food will usually come at a cost. That said, fresh fruit is almost always less expensive than packaged snack food. Milk is often less expensive than soda. While preparing quality food at home may be more expensive than grab-and-go fast food, quantifying the true cost of our nutritionally deficient diets—factoring in illness and health care costs—would almost certainly paint a different picture.

For years now we have been exporting our convenience-food culture to other nations, with predictable results. Thanks largely to its increase in American-style fast-food consumption, China now has the largest population of diabetics and pre-diabetics in the world, with a rate slightly higher than even the United States. Other non-communicable "lifestyle" diseases, such as heart disease, have also soared to U.S. levels. [2]

Acceptable Substitution

In the wellness industry, we use the terms "primary foods" and "secondary foods." Secondary foods are the macronutrients physically consumed, such as proteins, carbohydrates, fats, vitamins, and minerals. By contrast, primary foods are the tangible and intangible elements of our lives that influence the entirety of our health. These are things such as our social lives, relationships, home environments, careers, financial stability, and faith. When these primary foods are unbalanced, the predictable voids that are created are most often filled with food. As I say repeatedly to my clients, "It's not what you're eating, but rather what's eating you." Often, our consumption of food is an effort to compensate for something that's missing in the vocational, social, or spiritual spheres of our lives. This kind of eating can become reckless, even destructive, and only perpetuates the existing imbalances.

During my assessment sessions with new clients, I often see a light of recognition as an individual identifies an area of need. As we seek to balance these primary foods, we predictably see the secondary food issues begin to resolve.

Has food become an acceptable substitution for a primary food you lack? For love? Companionship? Stress relief? Accurately identifying voids in your life is the first important step toward taking control of your health. For those without a spiritual foundation, unbalanced behavior like this is understandable. For the follower of Christ, applying God's word will be the path to wholeness. The truths David presented in Chapter Seven can make all the difference for both the believer and the yet-to-believe.

Acute Habits

If I had to identify one activity that undermines nutritional integrity more than any other, bad habits would be it. I have counseled with countless clients whose progress toward good health is cannibalized by spontaneous snacking that is often associated with specific activities. Examples of this are the travelling salesman or truck driver who compulsively snacks on pork rinds or caramel popcorn clusters while driving, the sports junkie who has to shell roasted peanuts while watching ESPN, and the homemaker who has a weeknight ritual that includes a bowl of ice cream while watching the 10 o'clock news. Sometimes these binges replace meals, at other times they're reflexive add-ons. Regardless of their timing or nature, however, they are almost universally at odds with proper nutrition. It's amazing to consider how frequently nutritional balance is undermined by seemingly innocuous behaviors.

If you consume even 100 calories per day beyond what you burn through activity, you create a calorie surplus that will add ten pounds of body weight per year. What does 100 calories look like? Try nine chocolate-covered peanut candies or one-half of a sugary glazed donut. Making poor choices like these are why many Americans struggle with poor health. For the person intent on losing body fat, there are no inconsequential calories. Many of my clients justify poor eating habits by associating smaller portions with greater self-control. The reality is most are simply consuming more of these smaller portions translating to a greater caloric intake. The candy companies are not stupid. The proliferation of "bite-sized" offerings proves that marketers know people will snack all day on smaller portions, and end up consuming more than if they had eaten a regular-sized snack. So the "fun-size" is actually leading you to become a larger size.

Originally, I intended to include a list of "healthier" snacking options, but I would have only encouraged bad behavior. Our country is literally killing itself with its culture of snacking. The U. S. is the most overweight country, yet also the most undernourished. The vast majority of snacks are contributing nothing to the problem but empty calories. Soft chewy granola bars, portion-pack trail mixes, 100-calorie cracker packs, and the like are deceptive examples of snacks promising nutrition they can't deliver.

All calories are not created equal. Our body needs nutritionally dense calories, yet too often we supply it with calories void of nutrition. When our bodies are nutritionally deficient, the brain signals hunger regardless of calorie intake—increasing our desire to eat more. This physiological cycle perpetuates the destructive eating tendencies of habitual snackers.

For those who need nutritional coaching, I recommend finding a licensed nutritionist who can guide you toward new patterns of eating while helping you with your overall relationship with food. I am also available to help through our online services at *www.fit4theking.net*. As I've mentioned, however, taking an honest look at the six areas above and acting consistently in problem areas will resolve most nutritional issues.

Your body is an amazing, self-healing creation. It will respond to improved care and sustenance in remarkable ways. You owe it to yourself, your family, and your Creator to give your body what it needs need to not just survive—but to thrive!

1. "Dining Out on a Calorie Budget Nearly Impossible, Studies Find" by Liz Neporent. *Abcnews.go.com*, May 14, 2013.
2. "The Sick Man of Asia: China's Health Crisis" by Yanzhong Huang. *Foreign Affairs.*

CHAPTER 18

YOUR CALLING AS A STEWARD

"Moreover, it is required in stewards that one be found faithful"
1 Corinthians 4:2 (NKJV)

In 2007, the small Dutch community of Pella, Iowa, was abuzz with news that that development of a $150 million indoor rainforest was being considered near town. The enormous and unlikely undertaking was so grand in scope that, once it was built, it would become the largest attraction of its kind in the world, unseating the Eden Project located near London in Cornwall, England. Nearly overnight, people who hadn't spent one minute of their lives thinking about rainforests were catching EarthPark fever.

During that time, I was leading worship at a Pella church, so I had a ringside seat to the unfolding drama. Locations on a nearby reservoir were put forth, economic impact studies were commissioned, and side-project concepts started sprouting up like the tulips do in the town square each May. Plans included prairie grass preserves and sanctuaries for bonobos and other types of monkeys and apes.

The ecological euphoria that fell on the good folks of Marion County came courtesy of an acronym well-known in the investing community: OPM. When Other People's Money—in this case the U.S. taxpayers—was involved, the people of Pella set aside their famous cultural frugality. Big dreams were plentiful and no expense was considered excessive. When federal money was withdrawn, however, talk of a world-class arboretum disappeared as fast as a Dutch letter pastry at the town's annual heritage festival.

When other people's money is involved, we become very careless and spend-thrift. When our money is at stake, we're interested in getting the best value and results. Whether it's the biggest pastry or slice of pie from a bakery, we want to get our money's worth. We shop at sales for the best prices; we expect the most productivity from those we hire. We feel cheated when we learn we've missed a better value or paid people to remain idle. *It might surprise you to learn that God feels the same way about His investment in you and your body.*

Stewardship—not an option

We covered God's purposeful creation of us and learned that His end goal for His followers is not Heaven, but transformation into the likeness of Christ. A critical part of this transformation occurs when we stop viewing ourselves as owners and start seeing ourselves as God does: stewards. The word *steward* may sound dated or unfamiliar. *A steward is someone entrusted with another's wealth or property and charged with the responsibility of managing it in the owner's best interests.* [1]

According to the Bible, we're all stewards. We're responsible for our families, the material things we own, the intellectual capacity of our minds, and the physical capacity of our bodies. All these areas of our lives are on loan to us by God, who really holds the title to each of us. The only variable is how much we're entrusted with in these areas. Like any owner, He's looking for a return on His sizeable investment in each of us.

> *Don't you realize that your bodies are actually parts of Christ? ... You do not belong to yourself, for God bought you with a high price. So you must honor God with your body. 1 Corinthians 6:15,19,20 (NLT)*

Because God owns us, He can appropriately command us to love Him with our heart, soul, mind, and strength. His ownership is also the rationale behind our description of what it means to be *Fit For The King*.

> ***Being* Fit For The King *means being physically available to love God completely, let Him love others through you, and accomplish all He desires with you for His glory.***

Limiting our potential

Left to our own fleshly appetites and tendencies, many of us forget we're not in charge and allow our physical bodies to fall into disrepair. In so doing, we limit our functionality, vitality, and even our lifespan. Content with the notion that we've given our spirits over to the Lord, we forget that God expects us to offer our bodies to Him as well. *God's expectation of physical stewardship makes perfect sense, as the investments He makes in our spiritual growth can be neutralized or even lost prematurely when the physical body is not well cared for.*

Of what benefit are our spiritual gifts, our life experiences, our wisdom, or our testimonies when we are compromised by fatigue, illness, depression, or premature death? Pastors are especially susceptible to becoming unbalanced, if they forget to maintain the physical as well as the spiritual spheres of their lives. Pastor Pete Briscoe of Bent Tree Church in Dallas, Texas, nearly became a casualty of this kind of imbalance.

"I went a number of years without exercising. My health got really bad. The problem is I'm tall and slender, so I could hide it. I didn't put on 50 pounds and start to look overweight, but I was really unhealthy. My eating habits were terrible. I never exercised. I sat behind a desk for 20 years and just atrophied. I went to the doctor and had blood work done. I was pre-diabetic and my cholesterol was through the roof. The doctor said, 'We need some lifestyle changes. I don't see numbers like this in tall, slender guys like you.' I was on a dangerous path." [2]

Fortunately, Pastor Briscoe faced his issues and got help from his church leadership to address a potentially devastating snare to effective ministry. He realized that effectiveness in ministry and life was only possible when he owned the reality of stewardship and pursued health spiritually, mentally, and physically.

God's expectations defined

Like Pastor Briscoe, we have all experienced generous amounts of God's grace, mercy, patience, and forbearance in various shortcomings in our lives. Because of His kindness, it would be easy to view our Creator as one who's happy with anything we might choose to offer Him. We could build lives that focus on our pleasure and usurp His rightful ownership. This kind of mindset ignores God's understandable expectation for a "return" on His investment in us. Jesus presents this expectation vividly in a parable that describes both good and bad stewardship.

> *"Again, the Kingdom of Heaven can be illustrated by the story of a man going on a long trip. He called together his servants and entrusted his money to them while he was gone. He gave five bags of silver to one, two bags of silver to another, and one bag of silver to the last—dividing it in proportion to their abilities. He then left on his trip. The servant who received the five bags of silver began to invest the money and earned five more. The servant with two bags of silver also went to work and earned two more. But the servant who received the one bag of silver dug a hole in the ground and hid the master's money. After a long time their master returned from his trip and called them to give an account of how they had used his money. The servant to whom he had entrusted the five bags of silver came forward with five more and said, 'Master, you gave me five bags of silver to invest, and I have earned five more.' The master was full of praise. 'Well done, my good and faithful servant. You have been faithful in handling this small amount, so now I will give you many more*

responsibilities. Let's celebrate together! The servant who had received the two bags of silver came forward and said, 'Master, you gave me two bags of silver to invest, and I have earned two more.' The master said, 'Well done, my good and faithful servant. You have been faithful in handling this small amount, so now I will give you many more responsibilities. Let's celebrate together!' Then the servant with the one bag of silver came and said, 'Master, I knew you were a harsh man, harvesting crops you didn't plant and gathering crops you didn't cultivate. I was afraid I would lose your money, so I hid it in the earth. Look, here is your money back.' But the master replied, 'You wicked and lazy servant! If you knew I harvested crops I didn't plant and gathered crops I didn't cultivate, why didn't you deposit my money in the bank? At least I could have gotten some interest on it.' Then he ordered, 'Take the money from this servant, and give it to the one with the ten bags of silver. To those who use well what they are given, even more will be given, and they will have an abundance. But from those who do nothing, even what little they have will be taken away. Now throw this useless servant into outer darkness, where there will be weeping and gnashing of teeth.'
Matthew 25:14–30 (NLT)

We do great disservice to the message of this parable if we apply it merely to our finances. Jesus' ministry was focused on surrendered lives, not accumulating donors. His point is that we must use well what was given to us, including our physical bodies, which are significant matters of trust. Teaching in the "Olivet Discourse," Jesus warns future believers that we should watch for His return and order our lives accordingly. We should be "all in" for the Kingdom work He's given us—removing every hindrance and investing ourselves commendably should He arrive unannounced. Interestingly, those who are not concerned about life stewardship are condemned by the Master and chastised for preferring the diversion of food and drink to the assigned responsibilities of a steward (Matthew 24:49 and a parallel passage, Luke 12:45).

Examples of body stewardship

God has entrusted you with far more than financial resources. You must also exercise stewardship in regard to your spiritual gifts, time, intelligence capacity, relationships, and natural gifts. All of these can be mishandled or squandered by the way you act as steward of your life.

Of what benefit is a lifetime of walking with Christ if you're not available to disciple someone younger in the faith because you are fatigued? Have you robbed

God of needed service in His mission field due to physical constraints? If you were a competitive athlete, would you decline opportunities to serve because it interrupted your workout or dietary schedule? Do you decline service in the local church because you don't have the energy to be involved? Do you refuse to join in seasons of prayer and fasting because you can't conceive of denying yourself a meal or a week of meals?

Our congregation has been blessed with a parish nurse who has provided health information and assistance for many years. Several times a year, she travels internationally, sometimes to inhospitable countries, to teach, train, and equip national health-care workers who seek to serve others. These trips give her the opportunity to share a lifetime of medical knowledge and training, and also share the Gospel. This year she will travel to Thailand, Singapore, Chile, Honduras, and the Philippines to steward her gifts and knowledge. This dear lady turns 80 this year. She would be the first to tell you that she's been blessed with good health. It is also true that she has viewed her life as that of a steward, and that perspective has fueled years of Kingdom work.

A life like hers reminds me of Joshua and Caleb in the Old Testament. They had been obedient with a task given them, but many others were not. At roughly 40 years of age, both heard the regrettable news that, as punishment for those who had not obeyed, Joshua and Caleb along with Moses and all the people of Israel would spend the next 45 years roaming the desert. As a result of the failures of others, the two men wandered for four decades before they finally entered God's Promised Land. In light of this "life sentence," it would have been easy for them to set aside any sense of urgency regarding their future role or inheritance. Their perspective of stewardship and personal faith that God's promise was real, however, caused both to look 40 years into the future when their health, vigor, and experience would be sorely needed. They maintained their physical bodies in such a way that they could lead militarily into their eighties. As Caleb makes a request for his inheritance in the Promised Land of Canaan, the Bible records these amazing words:

> A delegation from the tribe of Judah, led by Caleb son of Jephunneh the Kenizzite, came to Joshua at Gilgal. Caleb said to Joshua, "Remember what the LORD said to Moses, the man of God, about you and me when we were at Kadesh-barnea. I was forty years old when Moses, the servant of the LORD, sent me from Kadesh-barnea to explore the land of Canaan. I returned and gave an honest report, but my brothers who went with me frightened the people from entering the Promised Land. For my part, I wholeheartedly followed the LORD my God. So that day Moses solemnly promised me, 'The land of Canaan on which you were just walking will be your grant of land and that of your descendants forever,

143

because you wholeheartedly followed the LORD my God.' Now, as you
can see, the LORD has kept me alive and well as he promised for all
these forty-five years since Moses made this promise—even while Israel
wandered in the wilderness. Today I am eighty-five years old. I am as
strong now as I was when Moses sent me on that journey, and I can still
travel and fight as well as I could then. So give me the hill country that
the LORD promised me. You will remember that as scouts we found the
descendants of Anak [giants] living there in great, walled towns. But if
the LORD is with me, I will drive them out of the land,
just as the LORD said." Joshua 16:4-12 (NLT)

At age eight-five, Caleb is tackling one of the hardest assignments in the conquest of the Promised Land. He's going to lead his clan against battle-hardened giants in walled cities—and prevail.

The Issue of personal responsibility

You may be thinking that God gave these people special provision for their tasks. That in His sovereignty, He appointed the years of their lives, and that nothing they did was going to interfere with that. While I wholeheartedly believe God knew the extent of their days, just as He knows yours and mine, God's sovereignty never overrides the necessity of our faith and obedience. After all, how many of their peers died in the "graves of craving" incident alone during their journey (Numbers 11)? Joshua and Caleb's vitality was a manifestation of the reward that faithful stewards receive.

"To those who use well what they are given, even more will be given,
and they will have an abundance. But from those who do nothing, even
what little they have will be taken away." Matthew 25:29 (NLT)

I don't know how many years God will give me. The fact that God knows, however, does not excuse me from being a faithful steward of the time, talents, treasure, and body He's given me. Rather than resign myself to a life of less-effective ministry, less-engaged family life, less-effective work as an employee, and fewer years to be engaged in all of these, I will follow the example of Paul when he states:

Don't you realize that in a race everyone runs, but only one person gets
the prize? So run to win! All athletes are disciplined in their training.
They do it to win a prize that will fade away, but we do it for an eternal

prize. So I run with purpose in every step. I am not just shadowboxing. I discipline my body like an athlete, training it to do what it should. Otherwise, I fear that after preaching to others I myself might be disqualified.
1 Corinthians 9:24-27 (NLT)

You won't find a greater proponent of God's sovereignty than Paul. Yet he is intent on giving his absolute best effort spreading the Gospel. Not a whiff of "God's going to get His job done regardless of my preparedness, effort, or longevity" here. From Paul's perspective, the stakes are so high he will give his best to the Kingdom work God entrusted to him. We continue the work today where eternal issues are at stake, and an expectant Master will be the final judge of our stewardship. A possible result of His evaluation, He makes clear, is a prize.

The Motivation Of Rewards

Does it feel somehow unseemly to be motivated to better stewardship by rewards? This incentive didn't seem to bother Paul. They were at the forefront of his mind and appear to be his consuming motivation, even to the conclusion of his ministry.

As for me, my life has already been poured out as an offering to God. The time of my death is near. I have fought the good fight, I have finished the race, and I have remained faithful. And now the prize awaits me— the crown of righteousness, which the Lord, the righteous Judge, will give me on the day of His return. And the prize is not just for me but for all who eagerly look forward to his appearing. 2 Timothy 4:6-8 (NLT)

No less than Moses and Jesus surrendered their own agendas to God's purposes with an eye to future rewards (Hebrews 11:26; 12:2).

Author Randy Alcorn helps put this in perspective:

"We must realize once and for all that the seeking of reward and the fulfilling of desires is not anti-Christian. What is anti-Christian is the self-centeredness that is unconcerned about God and one's neighbor, and the preoccupation with the immediate fulfilling of desires that distracts us from finding our ultimate fulfillment in Christ." [3]

I previously covered the unbiblical paradigm found so often in Western churches: Say a prayer, punch your ticket to Heaven, and live a self-obsessed life until God's (supposed) goal of getting you to Heaven becomes a reality. There is the assumption that Heaven is the great equalizer; that no matter how one has stewarded their resources, all will be treated exactly the same. If this was the case, why does Jesus go to such lengths to speak of stewardship, judgment, and rewards? Why has Paul reoriented his life around a passion for serving Christ well?

Dr. Alcorn, who has spent most of his life studying and writing about Heaven, speaks again to this issue when he writes:

"How dare we say that being in heaven is all that matters to us, when so much else matters to God? ... Scripture simply does not teach what most of us seem to assume—that heaven will transform each of us into equal beings with equal possessions and equal responsibilities and equal capacities. It does not say our previous lives will be of no eternal significance. It says exactly the opposite." [4]

Scripture is very clear that there is a heavenly correlation between what we invest here and experience there. It will not be the same for all (Proverbs 24:11-12; Matthew 19:27-30; Luke 14:12-14).

Given this reality, the initial distastefulness of stewarding our bodies through exercise, nutrition—and, yes, denial—is swallowed up in the prospect of generous reward for our discipline.

Then Jesus said to His disciples, "If anyone desires to come after Me, let him deny himself, and take up his cross, and follow Me. For whoever desires to save his life will lose it, but whoever loses his life for My sake will find it. For what profit is it to a man if he gains the whole world, and loses his own soul? Or what will a man give in exchange for his soul? For the Son of Man will come in the glory of His Father with His angels, and then He will reward each according to his works." Matthew 16:24-27 (NKJV)

"Well done, my good and faithful servant. You have been faithful in handling this small amount, so now I will give you many more responsibilities. Let's celebrate together!" Matthew 25:23 (NLT)

"And everyone who has left houses or brothers or sisters or father or mother or children or farms for My name's sake, will receive many times as much, and will inherit eternal life." Matthew 19:29 (NASB)

Perhaps our reward, celebration, and compound return will include the imperishable crown described in 1 Corinthians 9:24-25.

Alcorn writes again about the pursuit of difficult or counter-cultural goals as part of making sacrifices as a faithful steward:

"You still might not like it, though even that could change. But you would gladly do it in light of the promised rewards. Soldiers and athletes and farmers all know that short-term sacrifices are justifiable in light of their long-term benefits (2

Timothy 2:3-6). This is precisely the case for those who view eternity in proper perspective." [5]

Jesus' last words in Scripture begin with *"I am coming quickly and My reward is with Me, to give to everyone according to his work"* Revelation 22:12 (NKJV). The truth is, we were made to work for a reward. If we don't have our eyes on what Jesus promises, and pursue it with all our strength, we will settle for a lesser reward.

Judged And Rewarded

Inevitably the question of capacity will come up: "What about those who are physically or mentally handicapped? Will they be judged for their apparent lack of productivity?" Remember that God's concern was not the volume of gain that was generated by each steward, but by their attitude and faithfulness regarding what they had been given. Understanding that our lives are a gift from God to be fully invested for His glory is the point, not some arbitrary standard of physical perfection.

The late Dallas Theological Seminary professor Howard Hendricks was confronted with this issue of physical stewardship early in his ministry. Overweight as a young man, a mentor confronted him while he was attending seminary with the possibility that he was robbing God. Unsure what his mentor meant, Hendricks asked, "How am I robbing God?" His mentor basically said, *"The best years of your life, the years when you will have accumulated wisdom and experience and skill, you'll be in a grave instead of pouring your wisdom into young people when they'll really need it."*

Understanding the long-term Kingdom ramifications of his obesity, Hendricks made immediate adjustments to his lifestyle. Fit and trim through all his adult years, Hendricks left an undeniable legacy for the evangelical church when he passed away at the age of 88. It could be argued that the last twenty years of his ministry were the most fruitful.

Being a steward means asking hard questions: *Do I want to be fully engaged with my kids and grandkids? Do I want to possess the capacity to be enthusiastically involved in the vision of my local church? Do I want to meet my husband's or wife's needs as long as we both shall live? Do I want the freest years of my life to be spent "on mission" or in idle retirement, in a wheelchair, or in constant need of medical care because of my lifestyle decisions?*

Our wives, children, grandchildren, and friends will be impacted by our answers to these questions. More important, our Creator paid a high price for us and wants us to be passionate about giving Him the best return. After all, His creative capital is on the line.

1. The Grand Essentials by Ben Patterson, pg 7. Word, 1987.
2. Interview in Leadership Journal Winter/2014.
3. Money, Possessions and Eternity by Randy Alcorn, pg 168. Tyndale, 1989.
4. Ibid., pg 148-149.
5. Ibid., pg 133.

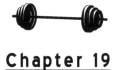

Chapter 19

Just Do It

When you've spent as much time in the gym as I have, you've heard and seen it all when it comes to fitness plans, workout regimens, insider tips, and bodybuilding apps. Fitness tools and methodologies are abundant, but it's perplexing why so few people consistently follow a plan that achieves the desired results. Most people don't have a plan because they thought the plan was simply obtaining a gym membership. Amidst a core of committed and experienced fitness enthusiasts, it's easy to become just another number cycling through the system.

If you hang around long enough, you will become familiar with this predictable cast of characters circulating in most fitness clubs:

- The Platehead, who cares only about pumping iron and whose muscles are so well developed that tying his or her shoes becomes nearly impossible;

- The Butter Churner, who spends an hour on the same piece of elliptical equipment every day until they're dripping with sweat;

- The Social Butterfly, who dresses the part but mostly exercises his or her jaw muscles;

- The One-Dimensional Lifter, who only uses the bench press and can be readily identified by protracted shoulders, pencil-thin legs, and arms that can't rotate;

- The Drifter, who randomly drifts from one piece of equipment to another;

- The Tourist, who drops his or her January membership by June after finding that the ten-minute facility tour they received when they signed up has done nothing to help them reach their fitness goal.

You want to avoid these stereotypes whenever possible. If only all the time, effort, and commitment consistently moved people toward better health and body function! Any time spent in a gym is of some benefit, but my desire is to help people accurately identify their health goals and take productive steps to see those goals realized.

Every client has needs and issues, a certain body type, and differing levels of interest, available time, and capacity for results. In the fitness world, one size does not fit all, which is why I'm not a fan of the typical industry approach to fitness I see displayed so pervasively in chain clubs. At the same time, I am a fan of utilizing a fitness center as you pursue a healthy lifestyle. There are a number of reasons.

1. Good fitness clubs provide a range of equipment, classes, and services. The staff usually includes personal trainers, who will assist you in developing a well-rounded fitness regimen that doesn't become stale, boring, or dangerously repetitive.

2. Help, supervision, and extra services are available so you learn, heal, and exercise safely.

3. Relationships can develop that not only provide accountability and encouragement, but also an opportunity to build redemptive relationships.

While pick-up basketball at the park, participation in a softball league, home video workouts, and home fitness equipment have their merits, these are not great long-term or exclusive fitness plans. It's in these scenarios that I see most injuries (competitive and repetitive), relapses (giving up), isolation, and lack of progress. These keep people from moving forward toward fitness goals. Most of these also lack the critical element of physiological progression, which helps you attain higher levels of fitness performance over time. Without this element, your body will stagnate, or plateau, and progress will be limited.

The role of a personal trainer—a role I've consistently played for over twenty-five years—is to identify goals, demystify equipment, guide workouts, provide a well-rounded fitness plan, and bring at least modest accountability to the table. Every person is different, so I customize schedules, workouts, meal plans, and such to maximize the results for each client.

It would be ludicrous for me to suggest a choreographed workout or routine for you to follow. These are the things I develop for my clients; they are specific for each person. There are, however, basic fitness principles that are applicable to all people as a foundation for productive time at the gym. If you are unfamiliar with fitness routines, equipment, or how to eat to maximize desired results, you will need a personal trainer for at least your first six to eight weeks.

Warming up/stretching

Warming up and stretching are the most commonly skipped steps in training—and the most common cause of injury in the gym. Especially critical if you are not active at home or work, the first ten minutes of any session should be spent on preparing your body for what's ahead. This will protect against muscle strain and tears, as well as get your heart rate elevated to an appropriate level for exercise. As little as six minutes at a relaxed pace on a treadmill or bike and four minutes of leg and upper body stretches can make a big difference in experiencing a pain-free and productive workout. (See stretching examples *www.fit4theking.net*)

Aerobics and resistance training

Anyone serious about becoming fit recognizes that they need to pursue cardio-vascular development. This can be done through such activities as running, biking, rowing, swimming, elliptical training equipment, or such strength development exercises as weight-lifting, isometrics, and working with bands. Too often, people gravitate toward what's familiar, easier, more enjoyable, or more accessible rather than developing a well-rounded fitness regimen. Some people combine cardio and resistance in their routines, others schedule cardio days and lifting days. Both approaches can work, but my experience leads me to favor incorporating both approaches in your fitness plan. By combining them, you don't miss a component when you can't exercise and this guards against overtraining in a particular area.

Anaerobic exercises are about strengthening your heart and lungs. Working to complete exhaustion isn't the goal, but if you're not perspiring at least moderately by the end of your workout, you should consider increasing the difficulty. This should comprise roughly thirty minutes of your workout. Here are some of the benefits of a cardiovascular workout:

— Rapid burning of calories (increased metabolism)

— Strengthening of heart and blood vessels

— Increasing capacity of lungs to oxygenate your blood (increased endurance)

— Improve flexibility and mobility of joints

David typically combines aerobic and resistance training in his workouts. Here are a typical week's cardio elements:

Sunday: Rest

Monday: Thirty minutes of brisk exercise on a stair-climber machine

Tuesday: Swim a variety of strokes for thirty minutes

Wednesday: Ride a spinning bike for thirty minutes (winter and windy days); ride a bike outside for sixty minutes (nice weather)

Thursday: Run on treadmill or outside for thirty minutes (three to four miles)

Friday: Thirty minutes on an elliptical machine

Saturday: Thirty to forty minutes on an elliptical machine or in an intense group aerobics class

Resistance training (lifting weights, etc.) is about increasing muscle mass, muscle flexibility, and muscle function. Resistance training holds benefits for both sexes, and not just the bodybuilder types. Muscle requires much more energy to function than fat or other tissue, so the more muscle you acquire, the more calories you will be burning—even in your sleep. Greater muscle mass will improve and aid in nearly everything you do, whether it be competitive or routine: gardening, working at a desk, running, riding in a car, carrying an infant, or climbing up stairs. Some of the many benefits of resistance training include:

- Increasing your capacity to burn calories (BMR)
- Increasing your capacity to function in all situations
- Increasing the flexibility of your ligaments and tendons
- Improving your posture
- Protecting your skeletal system
- Improving your confidence and appearance (symmetry in your physique)

The benefits of resistance training continue into your senior years, providing greater bone and muscle density, improved range of motion, and giving relief from arthritis pain.

Lifting all body parts

Talk to anyone who has adopted a weight-lifting routine, and you'll likely find they have certain days they anticipate and others they dread. Because of our body composition and other factors, we all tend to gravitate toward developing certain body parts at the expense of others. This can lead us to emphasize one particular group of muscles, which become well-developed while other muscle groups languish and atrophy. Anyone who's spent much time in a weight room has observed the guy with huge arms and a barrel chest whose pencil-thin legs rarely experience the leg press. Another scenario is the lifter who ignores his abdominal and back muscles, leaving him vulnerable to spinal and torso-related posture problems and injury. A protruding gut is a common for these lifters.

Getting huge biceps or a huge chest while ignoring other muscles can actually do more damage than not lifting at all. Unbalanced resistance training will, over time, move your arms, legs, neck, and torso out of their normal range of motion and set the stage for problems down the road, especially when you lift under-developed areas.

David's typical weekly resistance-training schedule is done in tandem with his cardio routine, which was listed above. You will notice that David tends to work opposing muscle groups on a couple of days.

Sunday: Rest

Monday: Thirty minutes of various abdominal exercises

Tuesday: Forty-five minutes of chest (front) and lats (back)

Wednesday: Thirty to forty minutes of various leg and gluteus (butt) exercises

Thursday: Thirty minutes of various shoulder exercises

Friday: Forty-five minutes of triceps (back of arm) and bicep (front of arm) exercises

Saturday: Catch up on muscle groups that he may have missed (or go to aerobics class)

The purpose of listing this is to show that David is working nearly all muscle groups each week, not to prescribe a workout for you. His routine is consistent with his goals (maintenance), his age, his schedule, injuries, etc. Working every muscle group each week may be unreasonable for you, and that's all right. The point is that rather than always heading for your favorite machine or barbell, mix up your routines and keep track of what you're working so you can keep it in balance. Again, this is where a personal trainer can be invaluable.

Our website is a great tool that provides visuals for building different muscle groups and organizing a sound lifting regimen. Check out some of our favorite lifts at *www.fit4theking.net.*

Recovery and muscle support

Following cardio work or resistance training, your body is hungry for nutrition that will help you recover the energy you've depleted and supply needed nutrients. This recovery and support can be accomplished through healthy food as well as supplements that are easily accessible online or through retailers. There are an exploding number of products coming to the market under the banner of workout aids, energy boosters, muscle support, and more, but we will not make recommendations because this area is fraught with potential dangers. There are, however, some basic practices and supplements you should be familiar with that will be of great benefit to you.

> **Build energy.** After a vigorous workout, rebuild muscle by drinking chocolate milk (skim or lowfat).
>
> **Use protein powder.** Use a meal replacement powder, ideally in a milk- or juice- based smoothie, within thirty minutes of a workout to provide your muscles what they need to rebuild and grow.
>
> **Stay well hydrated.** Drink water throughout your workout. As a daily routine, consume 75 to 125 fluid ounces of water (non-caffeinated and non-carbonated), depending on activity level and body weight. Keeping water available all day—regardless of thirst—is a must. Most people overeat due to dehydration, not hunger.
>
> **Application of deep-breathing techniques.** Muscle soreness after your workout should be expected, and breathing deeply from your diaphragm will help flush lactic acid, which has accumulated in your muscles, out of your system. This is an area where we could benefit from the experience of yoga practitioners.

Eating to support your goals

The key here is that you have identified a goal! Many people you see expending energy in a fitness center are living examples of Shakespeare's famous line from *Macbeth*—*"full of sound and fury, signifying nothing."* Despite their public efforts, their waistlines never shrink, their muscles never grow, their posture never improves, and they're always getting sick because their practices don't support lasting change. It's not that they are lackluster in their efforts, but as soon as they leave the gym they begin undoing the benefits of their workout. A good workout at the health club is a down payment toward good health, not a guarantee that gives someone the license to live recklessly once they leave the building.

Losing weight? Building muscle mass? Gaining endurance? Training for a specific sport? Lowering your LDL cholesterol? A combination of these? This is where a certified personal trainer with additional nutritional certifications can be of great benefit.

The default notion of dieting is that you need to eat less regardless of nutritional content. People think, "If I eat less, I'll lose weight." While there is some truth to this thinking, the short-term weight loss almost invariably ends a long-run weight gain. My Golden Rule in the area of nutrition is: *Don't diet, but eat with purpose. Eat more nutritious foods while consuming fewer calories.* You want to keep muscles performing and organs functioning while losing body fat. Simply eating less won't accomplish this and can sabotage future weight-loss goals.

Changing your routine

Our bodies have been created with an amazing ability to adapt to the stresses they encounter and restore balance. Many have heard the phrase "muscle has memory," and this truth is derived from this adaptive principle. When we fall into repetitive workout routines, we play to the body's adaptive ability which will eventually limit positive change. In the gym, we talk about the advantages of "confused progression" in our workouts. This sounds negative, but it is really a positive. A confused progression includes changes in the weight, repetitions, range of motion, machines or barbells utilized, exercises performed and intensity. The benefits of a confused state include a higher Basal Metabolic Rate (burning more calories), enhanced muscular function, and more rapid cellular repair.

In simple terms, this means that you will benefit from changing your workout routine on a regular basis. This applies to cardiovascular as well as resistance training. Again, this is where a fitness club and personal trainer can be of great benefit. He or she will have a variety of workout options for you, and any well-equipped heath center will have what you need to make your workouts interesting and productive.

Getting Started

As important as all I've covered so far is, here's the best advice I can give you: Don't let the ideal of a planned and organized fitness pursuit, the acquisition of a personal trainer, or a club membership keep you from getting started. Remember one thing: Start somewhere. Get in the game; don't stand on the sidelines. Everybody's fitness plan starts and ends with the same question: *What are you willing to do?*

— Are you willing to take the stairs, instead of the elevator?
— Are you willing to stand while you're on the phone?
— Are you willing to walk during your lunch break?
— Are you willing to pack a healthy lunch, instead of going for drive-thru?
— Are you willing to eliminate sugary drinks and sodas?

Get started and experience the benefits of positive change. As you see the first improvements in your body and overall well-being, my hope is you will strengthen your commitment to a fitness plan that will pay increasing dividends. At some point you will find yourself pursuing a fit lifestyle, rather than viewing it as a burden to be endured.

No Quick Fixes

You may notice in this chapter that I have not presented any quick fixes or ten-week plans. Fitness doesn't happen in ten weeks. Fitness is like spiritual growth. You can't microwave maturity or achieve instant physical change. Your unique fitness path will last a lifetime and involve successes, plateaus, and setbacks. It will be informed and inspired by the scriptural truths David has been presenting and, hopefully, aided and encouraged by some of the simple but powerful fitness principles I've shared here.

CHAPTER 20

YOUR CALLING AS AN AMBASSADOR

How beautiful on the mountains
are the feet of the messenger who brings good news,
the good news of peace and salvation,
the news that the God of Israel reigns!
Isaiah 52:7 (NLT)

Not many people ever meet, much less converse, with a U.S. ambassador. Because of friendships that stretch back to college, however, Beth and I have been able to personally witness the political rise of Mary Kramer, who was appointed by President George W. Bush to the ambassadorship to Barbados and the Eastern Caribbean from 2004 to 2006. For three years, Mary was the face of the United States to several million people, both pursuing our nation's interests as well as making it possible for people in the Caribbean region to access citizenship and educational opportunities available in our country. While serving, her character, demeanor, appearance, and language were on display daily, not simply as a reflection of herself, but as a reflection of the interests of the President.

God wants to be known, and He has used creation, His Word, and His followers to be the instruments through which His goodness and glory are communicated. Followers of Jesus are tasked with accurately representing Him to the world, even though some carry this like an unwanted burden. Christians cannot opt into or out of this responsibility, which is also true of our call to stewardship. If we are in Christ, we also have the privilege and responsibility of being His ambassador.

"So we are Christ's ambassadors; God is making his appeal through us.
We speak for Christ when we plead, "Come back to God!"
2 Corinthians 5:20 (NLT)

Trustees of the Gospel

Throughout history, God has appointed His people as "ministers of reconciliation." We take words of life to a world of confused people who operate under many false assumptions about who He is and about His love, care, and provision. We must accurately share the Good News of the Gospel to an unbelieving world in a winsome and engaging manner; one that removes any barriers to the message of the cross. Frankly, the cross will be enough of a barrier without our erecting others (1 Corinthians 1:18).

The ambassador gig has been fraught with trouble from the beginning. Adam and Eve, God's prototypes and first ambassadors, were seriously compromised shortly after their commissioning. The Jewish people largely fumbled their roles as ambassadors to the Gentiles (all non-Jews in the world). To move the leadership of the Early Church outside their comfort zone of Jerusalem, it took persecution. Only then did they take on the mantle of ambassadorship. Though God wants His people to take their critical roles in His Kingdom plans seriously, He is frequently met with resistance.

Looming even larger than our preparedness to quote Scripture is the fact that people are seeing the Gospel lived out in our daily lives through our conduct and appearance. From this perspective, what kind of gospel are they seeing and hearing from you?

The Apostle Paul was passionate about removing every barrier that might exist between him and a credible Gospel presentation:

> *Even though I am a free man with no master, I have become a slave to all people to bring many to Christ. When I was with the Jews, I lived like a Jew to bring the Jews to Christ. When I was with those who follow the Jewish law, I too lived under that law. Even though I am not subject to the law, I did this so I could bring to Christ those who are under the law. When I am with the Gentiles who do not follow the Jewish law, I too live apart from that law so I can bring them to Christ. But I do not ignore the law of God; I obey the law of Christ. When I am with those who are weak, I share their weakness, for I want to bring the weak to Christ. Yes, I try to find common ground with everyone, doing everything I can to save some. 1 Corinthians 9:19-22 (NLT)*

While it could be argued that conforming to cultural extremes of body care creates common ground with the rising number of unhealthy or body-obsessed people in this country, I'm not sure this is the spirit of Paul's message. We can create any number of common ground experiences with people, but only those that reflect a life pursuing Christ would be appropriate.

The Message And The Messenger

As a communications student at California State University, Fullerton, I was introduced to the philosophy of Canadian communication theorist Marshall McLuhan, originator of the term "global village." His theories were summarized in the famous phrase "The medium is the message," which means the *form of a medium embeds itself in the message, creating a symbiotic relationship by which the medium influences how the message is perceived.* In simple terms, there's no separating the message from the message-giver. Media gatekeepers have seized on this idea for the past half-century as they seek to deliver messages via credible spokespeople, appropriate venues, and relevant communication vehicles.

God has and will continue to use people of all different colors, shapes, and sizes to spread the Gospel. Jesus Himself said that He would build His church, and the gates of hell would not prevail against it (Matthew 16:18). At the time Jesus said this, there seemed to be only one disciple who had a clue as to what that program was. He knew that the Kingdom would move forward without regard to any obstacle. The question a conscientious ambassador would ask is, "Am I an obstacle?" Specific to the purposes of this book would be the questions, *"Is there something about my physical appearance that presents a barrier to anyone who needs to hear the Gospel?"* and *"Does my level of physical fitness allow me to feel vibrant and energized, so I can exude the joy that I claim Jesus has brought into my life?"*

Let's return again to our operating definition and goal statement.

Being* Fit For The King *means being physically available to love God completely, let Him love others through you, and accomplish all He desires with you for His glory.

When we seek to love others by allowing God to share the Gospel through our testimony, we are bringing more than Scripture verses to the table. *We are bringing the credibility of the transforming power of the Gospel as well.* We're going to share with our co-workers that God is love and that God loves us unconditionally. Do we look like we believe that? We're going to suggest that God has the power to remove addictions and compulsions that distort our lives. Do we look like we're walking in that power and self-control? We're going to read Scripture that informs our sin-weary friends that in Christ we are a "new creature" and that "old things have passed away and new things have come." Do we look like we're walking in the vibrant newness of life?

Asking these somewhat pointed questions is not intended to sabotage your efforts in personal evangelism, but it's a valuable exercise to do some personal evaluation of the "medium" when the message is so critical. It is absolutely true that we are all "jars of clay" and God uses flawed and simple people so, *"The excellence of the power may be of God and not of us" (2 Corinthians 4:7).* Yet a serious ambassador will take whatever steps necessary to assure the Gospel that people hear aligns with the Gospel that people see.

Jesus the Ambassador

When considering the ambassadors God has had represent Him before men, we have to look to Jesus as the prime example. Jesus claimed to be God in the flesh and invites all of us to follow Him in word, deed, and practice. Most of what we know about Jesus comes from the Bible, including some insight about His physical state.

We know from Isaiah that Jesus was not considered to be "handsome" in a way that would attract followers with sheer sex appeal.

> *"There was nothing beautiful or majestic about his appearance, nothing to attract us to him." Isaiah 53:2 (NLT)*

In describing the glory of God's physical presence among us, the Apostle John focuses on character, demeanor, and message.

> *"So the Word became human and made his home among us. He was full of unfailing love and faithfulness. And we have seen his glory, the glory of the Father's one and only Son." John 1:14 (NLT)*

There was no barrier to his developing physically and socially in ways that were in keeping with a good reputation and character.

> *"Jesus grew in wisdom and in stature and in favor with God and all the people." Luke 2:52 (NLT)*

His earthly father, Joseph, was a mason/carpenter by trade and Jesus followed in his footsteps. This work would develop and demand a strong physical body.

> *"Then they scoffed, 'He's just the carpenter's son, and we know Mary, his mother, and his brothers—James, Joseph, Simon, and Judas.'" Matthew 13:55 (NLT)*

At the outset of His public ministry, Jesus denied Himself food for forty days to concentrate on spiritual preparation for the work ahead of Him. He did not let a desire for physical ease, pleasure, meals, or a workout regimen take priority over spiritual matters (Luke 4:1-2).

Throughout his public ministry, Jesus traveled by foot over an area of hundreds of square miles. Every devout Jewish male went to Jerusalem three times per year to attend religious festivals. Since Jesus lived in Nazareth (and I think we can assume He was devout!), that would have been a 240-mile round-trip, three times per year. Between the ages of five and thirty, Jesus would have walked 18,000 miles in trips to Jerusalem alone (3 x 240 x 25).

It has been estimated that the total distance Jesus walked in His thirty-three years on earth was 21,525 miles. Here's how the distance was tallied:

- 400 miles from Egypt to Nazareth.

- 18,000 miles from Nazareth to Jerusalem and back by age thirty.

- 3,125 miles during His three-year public ministry. [1]

Burning calories was obviously not an issue for Jesus. But what about His food intake? He proved that He could produce food miraculously for Himself, His disciples, and others. And then there are all those instances of Jesus feasting with "gluttons and drunkards," such as at Matthew's house or with Zacchaeus (Luke 5:29, Matthew 11:19, Luke 19:1-11).

Despite recorded instances of his dining with people who had the means to provide a decent spread, this is not the norm we see portrayed in Scripture. Jesus and His disciples depended on the hospitality of generous followers or scavenged what they could from farm fields and they often bedded down on roadsides (Luke 6:1, Matthew 8:20). Given the picture of Christ's upbringing and the demands of His ministry, it's implausible to picture a chubby Jesus "living large" thanks to His ability to either coerce food and drink from his hosts or create food Himself. It should be noted that on the three occasions Jesus did miraculously transform or multiply food it was simple fare, consisting of dried fish, bread, or table wine.

He celebrated food in its proper context, as replenishment instead of indulgent consumption. He also reminded people that, as the Apostle Paul notes, the King-dom of God was not eating and drinking but pursuing the outflow of the Spirit in our lives (Romans 14:17).

Jesus was able to physically lead rugged younger fishermen and give compas-sionately to others despite what was often an incredibly demanding schedule of morning-to-evening ministry. He also set an example of prioritizing prayer and solitude as an energizing balance to His ministry workload (see example in Mark 1:16-39).

During the Passion, Jesus withstood the horrors of beatings, scourging, carrying His cross, and crucifixion in a manner that allowed God's complete work to be done.

Several times throughout Jesus' ministry, God the Father made it clear He was well pleased with the manner and spirit with which Christ obeyed and fulfilled His purposes (Matthew 3:17, 17:5, John 12:28-29).

What we see in Jesus, the ultimate Ambassador, is the embodiment of our guiding statement:

> *Being* **Fit For The King** *means being physically available to love God completely, let Him love others through you, and accomplish all He desires with you for His glory.*

It doesn't take beauty or charisma to please God and be an effective ambassador. Jesus shows us that obedience, availability, moderation, and fitness are all things we should aspire to as we seek to be instruments of God's glory.

Fit For Battle

Having lived on both sides of the physical and spiritual dimensions, Jesus possessed a unique perspective of spiritual warfare. He knew what He was up against and made spiritual and physical provision for His great task. It's safe to say that most of us give no thought to daily preparation of our bodies for spiritual warfare. Watchman Nee gives voice to this reality:

"...we should understand that the weariness which believers often experience in their body is in many respects distinct from that of ordinary people. Their consumption is more than physical. Because they walk with the Lord, bear the burdens of others, sympathize with the brethren, work for God, intercede before Him, battle the powers of darkness, and pommel their body to subdue it, food and rest alone are insufficient to replenish the loss of strength in their physical frame." [2]

Do we not understand that the follower of Christ has been called upon to perform double duty in their position as an ambassador? Ambassadors for Christ deal not only with the common physical realities that beset all people regardless of faith, but also the strength-sapping demands of spiritual combat.

> *"For our struggle is not against flesh and blood, but against the rulers, against the powers, against the world forces of this darkness, against the spiritual forces of wickedness in the heavenly places." Ephesians 6:12 (NASB)*

Can we fuel our physical bodies for this awesome task with highly processed foods and a sedentary lifestyle? We are in a spiritual battle and great demands are placed on ambassadors who are obediently engaged. In addition to preparing through spiritual disciplines, our physical and dietary habits need scrutiny as well.

When I think back to an incident during my teenage years, I'm reminded of spiritual realities. My father, a pastor, was rousted from a post-service nap one Sunday by a call from a family that had recently begun attending our church. Their daughter, whom my older brother and I knew from the high school we all attended, had gone on a bedroom-trashing tirade worthy of *The Exorcist.* They were convinced their daughter was demon possessed and were calling in reinforcements. Arriving at their home and confronting the situation, my dad quickly realized that the girl was possessed, indeed, and that the demon knew my dad and the purpose of his visit.

After the demon was cast out, she received Christ and, in the days following, related a hair-raising story of how her possession came about. The part of her story that always stuck with me was that the possessing demon told her specifically to "stay away from the Bush boys because they hate you." We did not know her well, and had no reason to hate her. But the demonic forces knew who we were, knew we were followers of Jesus, and viewed us as members of the opposing forces in a spiritual battle. This incident reminded us that the battle is real and ongoing—and we needed to stay prepared for it.

Boldness and confidence

When we think of an ambassador, we picture someone who is confident, engaging, and persuasive. One who, while being diplomatic, serves their leader with boldness. Is there anything about your appearance that saps your confidence? Any sense of embarrassment that keeps you from engaging others? Would it be correct to say that your witness for Christ has been muted or made irrelevant because of body issues that are within your power to correct? For the person who's physically fit, are your interactions with others centered around you and your figure? Are you fishing for compliments? Are people unable to see Jesus because they can't get past the persona you're trying to create?

Say It Like You Mean It

I'm still looking for a correlation
Between what you say and how you roll
Spit it out
Yeah, spit it out
Say it like you mean it
Say it like you mean it

Say it like you mean it
But I still don't believe it

Words and Music by Jon Foreman © 2013 Publishing Smublishing

Living as an ambassador for Christ is a daily awareness that, like it or not, we're called to rightly represent and give testimony to lives that are changed and controlled by the power of God's Spirit working in us. God could have chosen any number of ways to communicate His Gospel, but He has chosen us to be the communicators of His appeal to a new and better way of living. If we don't look like we're experiencing this ourselves, it's possible we're putting up barriers that don't have to be there. Let the Apostle Paul's words guide us as we reach out to those with whom God has given us proximity and influence.

"...according to my earnest expectation and hope, that I will not be put to shame in anything, but that with all boldness, Christ will even now, as always, be exalted in my body, whether by life or by death. For to me, to live is Christ and to die is gain."
Philippians 1:20-21 (NASB)

What Price Ambassadorship?

As you read about becoming winsome and credible ambassadors, you might ask where we draw the line on improving our bodies. Modern science and medicine have made it possible to reimagine our physical bodies in ways never thought possible. Hygienic routines that are daily habits for most of us today would have been considered luxuries fit for royalty 150 years ago. Where do we draw the line? What's for our own vanity and what's for the sake of the Kingdom?

Listed below are products, activities, and procedures that are available to most Americans today. I'm presenting them in a continuum that I believe reflects their purpose of health, hygiene, ambassadorship, vanity, and body obsession. Move through this list and make a note of where you'd "draw the line" for an ambassador of Christ. In your opinion, what things are important or necessary to be a relevant and engaging vessel for the Gospel in our culture? What things only appeal to cultural expectations or our own vanity and desire to conform?

Deodorant

Toothpaste

Posture

Appropriate BMI (healthy weight/height proportionality)

Lasik vision correction

Hairstyle and color treatments

Cosmetics

Manicures and pedicures

Orthodontics (braces for your teeth)

Fashionable clothes

Facials

High level of physical fitness (more of a sculpted body)

Teeth whitening

False eyelashes

Colored contact lenses

Tanning

Laser hair removal

Microdermabrasion/chemical peel

Eyelid surgery (lifting)

Body piercing and tattoos

Hair grafts/hair regrowth medications

Botox

Breast augmentation, post-nursing

Liposuction/tummy tuck

Collagen injections

Facelift/necklift

Breast implants/pectoral implants

Anabolic steroids

This is not an exhaustive list, but you get the idea. Sincere ambassadors will draw lines in different places. In a culture that spares no expense to preserve a youthful appearance, however, ambassadors do well to remember that we are serving at the pleasure of an audience of One. First and foremost we are representing His Kingdom, not building one of our own.

"But we have this treasure in earthen vessels, so that the surpassing greatness of the power will be of God and not from ourselves…"
2 Corinthians 4:7 (NASB)

God designed our bodies to live forever, so the internal longing to perpetuate our youth and forestall death is a natural one. But because we are polluted with sin, this longing will only be fulfilled in Heaven. Our attempts to sustain a youthful persona via surgery and drugs may actually send a message that this world and this life are of paramount importance and worth clinging to at any cost. The fact is we are ambassadors of a different Kingdom, one that longs for redemption and consummation in Jesus that will only be completely fulfilled in His presence.

Since we are all appointed to represent Him, His interests, and His Kingdom, we must take our ambassadorships seriously and remove any barriers so those who do not know Jesus can see Him through us.

1. The estimate used here of the number of miles Jesus walked during his lifetime is published widely on the Internet, however an extensive search did not turn up the name(s) of the researcher(s) who made the original calculations.
2. *The Spiritual Man* by Watchman Nee. Living Stream Ministry, 1992.

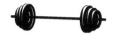

CHAPTER 21

PRIDE AND PREJUDICE

Today I quit my job. After twenty-five years in the fitness industry, I finally hit a wall I could no longer scale, dig under, or navigate around. My reasons for walking away are numerous and varied: I'm underpaid and under-respected, the hours are not conducive to a stable family life, and after owning a gym, it's hard working with people who have a different vision.

Mostly, though, I'm tired of lying to many of my clients. Not literally lying, but not telling the whole truth—the most important and relevant truth they need to hear. I care deeply about those I serve and I want to give them the information and inspiration they need to reach their goals and enjoy fuller, more productive lives. For many years I've committed myself to this and have enjoyed unusual success that has continued to fuel my fire. Increasingly, however, I feel like I'm fighting a holistic health battle with one hand tied behind my back. While boiler-plate cheerleading and workout regimens produce results for many, an increasing number of my clients need spiritual medicine I'm not allowed to dispense. And that barrier has convicted and convinced me that I'm engaged in transformational malpractice.

So I've retreated to a local coffee house for a dark roast while I try to talk myself off the vocational ledge I've just constructed. I absent-mindedly adjust the java jacket on my cup when I realize there's a message on the jacket calling for my attention. Reading the verbiage, I see I'm being invited to "Steep My Soul" by taking a quiet moment to reflect and collect my thoughts. To guide me in this exercise is a quote from Oprah Winfrey, who steeps a lot of souls: *"Be more splendid. Be more extraordinary. Use every moment to fill yourself up."*

As a follower of Jesus—and because I know the brand of spirituality Oprah is peddling—I immediately dismiss this entreaty as being deceivingly subtle, wrongly focused, and unbiblical. I mean, any advice coming from a coffee megachain and Oprah has got to be wrong … right? Yet isn't this essentially the message I share with my clients day after day? A message of unquestioning optimism, encouragement, positivity, and potential? A message that, without a proper context, I refuse to share anymore.

The Importance Of A Biblical Context

Being a fitness coach often means being a cheerleader. I look for potential in people they cannot see themselves. I'm an instiller of dreams, goals, and possibilities that have long been dead and forgotten. My job is moving someone past mental, emotional, and physical barriers that keep them locked out of full participation in their work, their families, and their world. I have a toolbox full of best practices, proven methods, silver bullets, and motivational jargon designed to unlock individual potential and usher in a new way of living. Increasingly, however, I feel convicted that a prejudice against spiritual truth leaves the most effective tools in the box.

In all honesty, I'm endeavoring to develop in my clients *a healthy, biblical pride in who they are and what they can accomplish with God's grace and strength.*

In the Old Testament, we read:

> *"For you formed my inward parts;*
> *you knitted me together in my mother's womb.*
> *I praise you, for I am fearfully and wonderfully made.*
> *Wonderful are your works; my soul knows it very well."*
> *Psalm 139:13-14 (ESV)*

And every competitor's favorite verse:

> *"For I can do everything through Christ, who gives me strength."*
> *Philippians 4:13 (NLT)*

These and other treasures from God's Word provide a platform for respect, dignity, pride, hope, endurance, patience, aspiration, and transformation. Think of all we gain from the Bible verses.

- They give us a rationale for getting up and starting over again when we fail and have every (human) reason for giving up on ourselves.

- They give us a right to feel proud about how we look and feel when we have achieved our goals.

- They give us a reason to praise the One who has granted us the opportunity to pursue a balanced, counter-cultural approach to health and fitness.

My current dilemma is this: Without a biblical framework to motivate my clients, *and the freedom to tell them the whole truth,* I'm left with nothing more than self-centered cheerleading that offers no more Truth than the ethereal musings on my coffee cozy.

"You can do it, Suzy, you're worth it! " (Says who?)

"You're getting totally ripped, dude!" (For whom?)

"This class is going to change your life!" (For what purpose?)

Without question, helping lead people toward a life of greater dignity and productivity is a worthwhile endeavor. But devoid of the Gospel, it can perpetuate self-centered and prideful motivations, which are the root of our sinful condition.

While my training business is on hold, I will be working with David on this book, creating an online coaching presence through *www.transformation-U,* developing *Inspire* health conferences that espouse a biblical fitness and nutrition perspective, and investigating a church-based fitness and recreation ministry.

In the midst of my own broken dreams, postponed aspirations, uncertain future, and professional frustration, I will have an opportunity to test the truth of what I've been longing to openly tell my clients for the eight years I've been walking with Jesus: *God loves you and proved it at Calvary. You are His idea. You're created to glorify Him. He owns everything and is sovereign over everything. No experience is wasted when you're submitted to God's purposes. All of this ends well.*

Put that on a coffee cup.

CHAPTER 22
THE LOVE REVOLUTION

It was 6 a.m. and I was sobbing uncontrollably. My face was buried in the family room sofa where I knelt praying in the predawn darkness. Concluding a season of prayer and fasting, I was unusually grieved at the reflection of Jesus that the Church portrayed to a lost culture. In the opinion of most of the lost, anyone bearing the name of Christ is judgmental, legalistic, homophobic, disengaged, hypocritical, and mostly motivated by political power. A true heart cry was rising from me, forming as a dangerous question: *We are so messed up ... forgive us... forgive me ... what does a follower of Jesus do to show Your true heart to lost people?*

With clarity I had never experienced before or since, God spoke an answer to my heart:

If you want to know my heart for lost people, here's someone you should pursue with the purpose of meeting his needs. He's black. He's gay and HIV positive. He's from the inner city. He's dying and he needs your help.

Overwhelmed by this download of information, I wondered in the weeks that followed what it meant. I didn't know anyone like this. How would I find him? What kind of help did he need? I considered shrugging it off as some kind of spiritual miscue, but the message continued to pervade my thoughts and prayers. I reaffirmed to God that I was willing to cooperate, but needed more information.

It was a Saturday when the puzzle started getting pieced together. I was reading the morning paper when my eyes travelled to a small sidebar that lamented the closing of a restaurant in Des Moines' inner city area. Its owner, a young black man, was experiencing undisclosed health problems and was shutting down. Near the end of the article it mentioned his involvement with the local gay community through the LGBT Resource Center. I felt an immediate confirmation from God's Spirit. *This is the man I've been telling you about.*

An awkward call to the Resource Center followed, where I left my name and number. A day later J. C. called me back and agreed to meet for breakfast. Thus began a transformative two-year relationship that included numerous meals together (including some the partner with whom J.C. lived), visits to J.C.'s home, workouts and tennis matches at the local club (he wanted me to be his doubles partner for the Gay Games!). There were also evening visits to the hospital dialysis center, where impurities were removed from his blood due to his failing kidneys.

As we became closer, I was able to share with him (and his partner) about my faith in Christ and what animated my life, including my serious pursuit of fitness. J. C. began to share with me about his declining quality of life, his broken family relationships, his questions about God, and his desire to be enrolled in a special new medical program that could open the door to a much-needed kidney transplant. As my wife had recently been a kidney donor for her father, I understood with unusual clarity all that was involved with this pursuit.

What was involved for a donor was lots of testing and type-matching, lots of in-convenience, invasive surgery, recovery, missed work, pain, scars, and, ultimately, the loss of one of the donor's two kidneys. I understood what God was asking me to consider, but to be honest this didn't align well with my health plans and goals. Why should I even entertain the thought of meeting his physical need? All that potential pain and inconvenience for a gay black man who was only living with the consequences of his chosen lifestyle? One who hadn't yet shown a willingness to repent?

When J. C. excitedly shared with me that he had been accepted into a first-of-its-kind transplantation program at the University of Minnesota, I felt it was time to share more about my pursuit of a relationship with him than I had previously.

An unforgettable lunch meeting followed at which I shared the prayer and God's answer that had brought us together nearly a year earlier. I told J. C. that God told me what he'd only shared with his partner—that he was HIV positive—and that I understood why a transplant was a long shot for him. Then I told him that I was submitting my name to be his kidney donor through the Minnesota program. Tears came to his eyes as he tried to comprehend not only my offer, but also the fact that God knew all about him, loved him, and was possibly making provision through me for his greatest physical need.

Months of testing, physical and emotional evaluations, and trips to Minnesota followed. But the suspense ended abruptly when a slightly elevated creatinine level in my final blood workup was flagged as a reason to remove me as a donor candidate.

After hearing this news, I visited a local nephrologist to see if I was in any danger. After telling him about the transplantation program and my removal from consideration, my doctor gave a resigned nod. "I'll take your kidney today," he said. "Your creatinine level is nothing more than a reflection of your muscle mass and is completely healthy and expected. You need to understand that they were looking for a reason to get you out of that program, and your blood test gave them just enough of a reason to do it. You would have been the first kidney transplant to an HIV-positive donor in history, and I'm sure they want to run a trial with a cadaveric kidney first before they risk wasting a kidney from a live donor who's not a perfect match."

To be honest, I was confused and a little devastated. I thought the end game was a grand gesture of selflessness that would publically illustrate God's love for lost people. What God apparently desired was a *relationship* made possible by a surrendered heart and available body.

J.C.'s health continued to deteriorate, and he found it necessary to move to a southern state, where the climate was not so hard on his compromised immune system. I have not heard from him for several years now.

The purpose of this story from my life is not to draw attention to myself, sensationalize my walk with God, or even suggest that this is the standard Jesus will expect of all His followers. It is, however, an example of the practical actions that flow from a life and a physical body that is stewarded for Kingdom purposes. It represents the kinds of love-motivated actions an ambassador would consider pursuing when they felt God's leading. It illustrates an intentional act of *worship* that surrenders everything to the One who's worthy of all we are.

This bodily surrender of worship occurs anytime we set aside the culturally-conforming impulse to make more of ourselves or less of our bodies than God does. It occurs anytime we are motivated by serving God and others more than we are by fleshly gratification. Like all true worship, it costs us something.

Let's return one last time to our definition statement:

***Being* Fit For The King** *means being physically available to love God completely, let Him love others through me, and accomplish all He desires with me for His glory.*

If my life had been characterized by an unhealthy relationship with food leading to poor health, I never would have put myself in a position of fasting so I could more clearly hear from God. And I certainly wouldn't have become a realistic donor candidate. My own health would have been so fragile I wouldn't have even been considered.

On the other hand, if my life were consumed with a pursuit of physical perfection and guarding my own health at all costs, I would never have stepped forward to love God and someone He wanted to touch through me.

God is calling us to glorify Him in our bodies through daily, worshipful surrender. Big and small steps of obedience are the fruit of that settled question of ownership.

I began this book with a call to revolutionary thinking regarding our physical bodies. Perhaps the need for revolutionary thinking in this area seemed contrived or overstated when you first read it. As you come to the end, however, perhaps the countercultural nature of our battle is hitting home. Within and without the walls of the church, we experience the relentless pull of cultural extremes and a daily spiritual battle that carries a very real cost.

Our Love Revolution is worth all this and more. Our husbands and wives, our children and grandchildren, and a world desperately seeking examples of authentic transformation will all be touched by our reasonable worship. In the end, however, the life that will have been transformed the most will be your own.

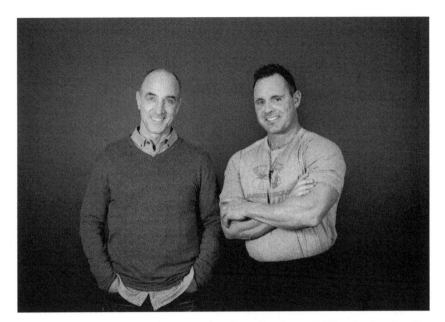

David Bush is an Iowa transplant, moving from Southern California shortly after marrying Beth, his wife of twenty-seven years. After stints in hospital management and developing a regional ice cream company, David moved into church-based ministry pursuits. A singer, songwriter and worship leader, David has shared his music with radio and live audiences across the country. While he has recorded four full projects of original material, *Fit For The King* is David's first book. A father of four boys, David continues to lead worship at his home church in Des Moines, Iowa while developing health, fitness and nutrition seminars and conferences.

Joe Tewell is a certified fitness trainer and licensed wellness coach with 25 years of experience in the fitness industry. He has managed and owned health clubs in Greater Kansas City and Des Moines in addition to working with both professional and high school sports teams. Recently Joe formed his own personalized wellness company, Transformation-U, which teaches the behaviors of healthy living. Joe and his wife Angel reside in Pleasant Hill, Iowa with children Marie and James.

67128517R00100

Made in the USA
Columbia, SC
27 July 2019